EXPERT **LPN** GUIDES

ECG
Interpretation

EXPERT LPN GUIDES

ECG Interpretation

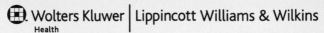

Wolters Kluwer | Lippincott Williams & Wilkins
Health

Philadelphia · Baltimore · New York · London
Buenos Aires · Hong Kong · Sydney · Tokyo

STAFF

EXECUTIVE PUBLISHER
Judith A. Schilling McCann, RN, MSN

EDITORIAL DIRECTOR
H. Nancy Holmes

CLINICAL DIRECTOR
Joan M. Robinson, RN, MSN

ART DIRECTOR
Elaine Kasmer

EDITORIAL PROJECT MANAGER
Christiane L. Brownell, ELS

EDITOR
Louise Quinn

COPY EDITORS
Kimberly Bilotta (supervisor), Tom
DeZego, Jen Fielding, Shana
Harrington, Dorothy P. Terry,
Pamela Wingrod

DESIGNER
Jan Greenberg

DIGITAL COMPOSITION SERVICES
Diane Paluba (manager), Joyce Rossi
Biletz, Donna S. Morris

MANUFACTURING
Beth J. Welsh

EDITORIAL ASSISTANTS
Megan L. Aldinger, Karen J. Kirk,
Linda K. Ruhf

INDEXER
Dianne Schneider

LPNECG010307

Library of Congress Cataloging-in-Publication Data

LPN expert guides. ECG interpretation.
    p. ; cm.
  Includes bibliographical references and index.
  1. Electrocardiography—Handbooks, manuals, etc. 2.
Nursing—Handbooks, manuals, etc. I. Lippincott Williams & Wilkins. II. Title: ECG interpretation.
  [DNLM: 1. Electrocardiography—nursing—Handbooks. 2. Nursing, Practical—methods—Handbooks. WY 49 L9234e 2007]
  RC683.5.E5L76 2007
  616.1'207547—dc22   2006100517
  ISBN-13: 978-1-58255-701-4 (alk. paper)
  ISBN-10: 1-58255-701-2 (alk. paper)

Contents

Contributors and consultants

Penny S. Bennett, RN, BSN
Surgical Unit Charge Nurse
Good Shepherd Health System
Longview, Tex.

Linda J. Franklin, RN, AA, BSN
Practical Nursing Instructor
Meridian Technology Center
Stillwater, Okla.

Donna Halloran-Krol, RN, BSN
Assistant Professor
Ivy Tech Community College
Valparaiso, Ind.

Michelle Johnson, RN, BSN
Assistant Professor
Northern Michigan University
Marquette

Janis Simpson, RN, BSN, MA, Eds
Nursing Coordinator
Tennessee Technology Center
Athens

Gina Sirach, RN, MSN
Nursing Faculty
Southeastern Illinois College
Harrisburg

Beverly Skloss, RN, MSN
Coordinator of Student Development
Valley Baptist Medical Center School of Vocational Nursing
Harlingen, Tex.

Audrey E. Taleff, APRN,BC, MSN
Family Nurse Practitioner
Waianae (Hawaii) Coast Comprehensive Health Center

1

CARDIAC ANATOMY AND PHYSIOLOGY

With a good understanding of electrocardiograms (ECGs), you'll be better able to provide expert care to your patients. For example, when you're caring for a patient with an arrhythmia or a myocardial infarction, an ECG waveform can help you quickly assess his condition and begin lifesaving interventions.

To build ECG skills, begin with the basics covered in this chapter—an overview of the heart's anatomy and physiology.

Cardiac anatomy

The heart is a hollow muscular organ that works like a mechanical pump. It delivers oxygenated blood to the body through the arteries. When blood returns through the veins, the heart pumps it to the lungs to be reoxygenated.

LOCATION AND STRUCTURE
The heart lies obliquely in the chest, behind the sternum in the mediastinal cavity, or mediastinum. It's located between the lungs and in front of the spine. The top of the heart, called the *base*, lies just below the second rib. The bottom of the heart, called the *apex*, tilts forward and

Where the heart lies

The heart lies within the mediastinum, a cavity that contains the tissues and organs separating the two pleural sacs. In most people, two-thirds of the heart extends to the left of the body's midline.

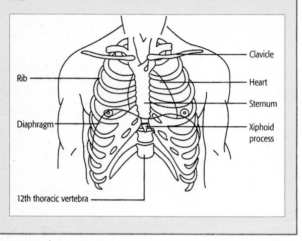

down toward the left side of the body and rests on the diaphragm. (See *Where the heart lies*.)

LIFE STAGES *An infant's heart is positioned more horizontally in the chest cavity than an adult's heart. As a result, the apex is at the fourth intercostal space. Until age 4, the apical impulse is to the left of the midclavicular line. By age 7, the heart is located in the same position as the adult heart.*

The heart varies in size, depending on the person's body size, but is roughly 5″ (13 cm) long and 3¾″ (9.5 cm) wide, or about the size of a fist. The heart's weight, typically 9 to 12 oz (255 to 340 g), varies depending on the person's size, age, gender, and athletic conditioning.

An athlete's heart usually weighs more than average, and an elderly adult's heart weighs less.

◗ *LIFE STAGES As a person ages, his heart usually becomes slightly smaller and loses its contractile strength and efficiency. By age 70, cardiac output at rest has diminished by 30% to 35% in many people.*

HEART WALL

The heart wall is made up of three layers:

■ The epicardium, the outermost layer, is made of squamous epithelial cells overlying connective tissue.
■ The myocardium, the middle and thickest layer, is the largest portion of the heart's wall and contracts with each heartbeat.
■ The endocardium, the heart wall's innermost layer, is a thin layer of endothelial tissue that lines the heart valves and chambers. (See *Layers of the heart wall,* page 4.)

PERICARDIUM

The pericardium is a fluid-filled sac that envelops the heart and acts as a tough, protective covering. It consists of the fibrous pericardium and the serous pericardium. The fibrous pericardium is made of tough, white tissue, which fits loosely around the heart and protects it. The serous pericardium, the thin, smooth, inner portion, has two layers:

■ the parietal layer, which lines the inside of the fibrous pericardium
■ the visceral layer, which adheres to the surface of the heart.

The pericardial space separates the visceral and parietal layers and contains 10 to 20 ml of thin, clear pericardial fluid that lubricates the two surfaces and cushions the heart.

Layers of the heart wall

This cross section of the heart wall shows its various layers.

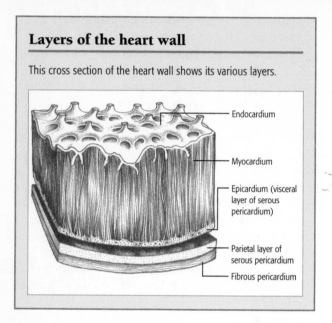

- Endocardium
- Myocardium
- Epicardium (visceral layer of serous pericardium)
- Parietal layer of serous pericardium
- Fibrous pericardium

CHAMBERS OF THE HEART

The heart contains four chambers—two atria and two ventricles.

Atria

The right atrium lies in front of and to the right of the smaller but thicker-walled left atrium. An interatrial septum separates the two chambers and helps them contract. The right and left atria serve as volume reservoirs for blood being sent into the ventricles. The right atrium receives deoxygenated blood returning from the body through the inferior and superior venae cavae and from the heart through the coronary sinus. The left atrium receives oxygenated blood from the lungs through the four pulmonary veins. The contracting atria forces blood into the ventricles.

Ventricles

The right and left ventricles are the pumping chambers of the heart. The right ventricle lies behind the sternum and forms the largest part of the heart's sternocostal surface and inferior border. The right ventricle receives deoxygenated blood from the right atrium and pumps it through the pulmonary arteries to the lungs, where it's reoxygenated. The left ventricle forms the heart's apex, most of its left border, and most of its posterior and diaphragmatic surfaces. The left ventricle receives oxygenated blood from the left atrium and pumps it through the aorta into the systemic circulation. The interventricular septum separates the ventricles and helps them pump.

Chamber wall

The amount of pressure needed to eject blood determines the thickness of a chamber's walls. Because the atria act as reservoirs for the ventricles and pump the blood against a lower pressure, their walls are considerably thinner than the walls of the ventricles. Likewise, the left ventricle has a much thicker wall than the right ventricle because the left ventricle pumps blood against the higher pressures in the aorta. The right ventricle pumps blood against the lower pressures in the pulmonary circulation.

HEART VALVES

The heart contains four valves—two atrioventricular (AV) valves (tricuspid and mitral) and two semilunar valves (aortic and pulmonic). Each valve consists of cusps, or leaflets, that open and close in response to pressure changes within the chambers they connect. The primary function of the valves is to keep blood flowing forward through the heart. When the valves close, they prevent backflow, or regurgitation, of blood between chambers.

The sounds of the valves closing make up the heart sounds.

AV valves

The two AV valves located between the atria and ventricles are:

■ the tricuspid valve, named for its three cusps, which separates the right atrium from the right ventricle

■ the mitral valve, sometimes referred to as the bicuspid valve because of its two cusps, separates the left atrium from the left ventricle.

The closing AV valves make the S_1, or the first heart sound.

The cusps, or leaflets, of these valves are anchored to the papillary muscles of the ventricles by small tendinous cords called *chordae tendineae*. The papillary muscles and chordae tendineae work together to prevent the cusps from bulging backward into the atria during ventricular contraction. Disruption of either of these structures may prevent valves from closing completely, allowing blood to flow backward into the atria. This backward blood flow may cause a heart murmur.

Semilunar valves

The semilunar valves, so called because their three cusps resemble half moons, are:

■ the pulmonic valve, located where the pulmonary artery meets the right ventricle, which permits blood to flow from the right ventricle to the pulmonary artery and prevents backflow into the right ventricle

■ the aortic valve, located where the left ventricle meets the aorta, which allows blood to flow from the left ventricle to the aorta and prevents blood backflow into the left ventricle.

Increased pressure within the ventricles during ventricular systole causes the pulmonic and aortic valves to open, ejecting blood into the pulmonary and systemic circulation. Loss of pressure as the ventricular chambers empty causes the valves to close. The closing of the semilunar valves makes the S_2, or the second heart sound.

BLOOD FLOW THROUGH THE HEART

Understanding the flow of blood through the heart is critical for understanding the overall functions of the heart and how changes in electrical activity affect peripheral blood flow. It's also important to remember that right and left heart events occur at the same time. (See *Inside a normal heart,* page 8.)

Deoxygenated blood from the body returns to the heart through the inferior vena cava, superior vena cava, and coronary sinus and empties into the right atrium. The increasing volume of blood in the right atrium raises the pressure in that chamber above the pressure in the right ventricle. Then, the tricuspid valve opens, allowing blood to flow into the right ventricle.

The right ventricle pumps blood through the pulmonic valve into the pulmonary arteries and lungs, where oxygen is picked up and excess carbon dioxide is released. From the lungs, the oxygenated blood flows through the pulmonary veins and into the left atrium. This completes a circuit called *pulmonary circulation.*

As the volume of blood in the left atrium increases, the pressure in the left atrium exceeds the pressure in the left ventricle. The mitral valve opens, allowing blood to flow into the left ventricle. The ventricle contracts and ejects the blood through the aortic valve into the aorta. The blood is distributed throughout the body, releasing oxygen to the cells and picking up carbon dioxide. Blood

Inside a normal heart

This cross section shows the internal structures and blood flow to and from the heart.

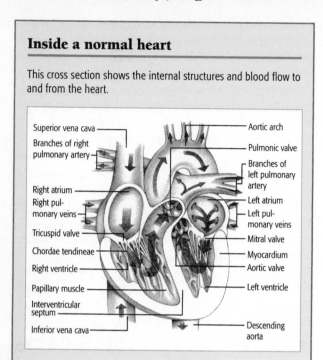

Superior vena cava

Branches of right pulmonary artery

Right atrium

Right pulmonary veins

Tricuspid valve

Chordae tendineae

Right ventricle

Papillary muscle

Interventricular septum

Inferior vena cava

Aortic arch

Pulmonic valve

Branches of left pulmonary artery

Left atrium

Left pulmonary veins

Mitral valve

Myocardium

Aortic valve

Left ventricle

Descending aorta

then returns to the right atrium through the veins, completing a circuit called *systemic circulation.*

CORONARY BLOOD SUPPLY

Like the brain and all other organs, the heart needs an adequate supply of oxygenated blood to survive. The main coronary arteries lie on the surface of the heart, with smaller arterial branches penetrating the surface into the cardiac muscle mass. The heart receives its blood supply almost entirely through these arteries. In fact, only a very small percentage of the heart's endocardial surface can obtain sufficient amounts of nutrition directly from the

Vessels that supply the heart

The coronary circulation is the arterial system of blood vessels that supply oxygenated blood to the heart and the venous system that removes oxygen-depleted blood from it.

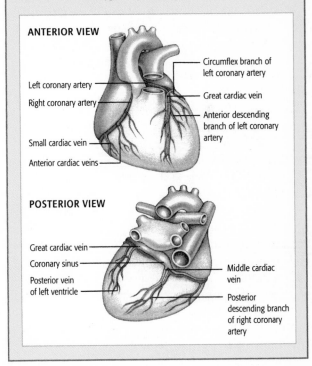

ANTERIOR VIEW

Circumflex branch of left coronary artery

Left coronary artery

Right coronary artery

Great cardiac vein

Anterior descending branch of left coronary artery

Small cardiac vein

Anterior cardiac veins

POSTERIOR VIEW

Great cardiac vein

Coronary sinus

Posterior vein of left ventricle

Middle cardiac vein

Posterior descending branch of right coronary artery

blood in the cardiac chambers. (See *Vessels that supply the heart*.)

Understanding coronary blood flow can help you provide better care for a patient with coronary artery disease because you'll be able to predict which areas of the heart would be affected by a narrowing or occlusion in a particular coronary artery.

Coronary arteries

The left main and right coronary arteries arise from the coronary ostia, small orifices located just above the aortic valve cusps. The right coronary artery fills the groove between the atria and ventricles, becoming the acute marginal artery and ending as the posterior descending artery. The right coronary artery supplies blood to the:

- right atrium
- right ventricle
- inferior wall of the left ventricle
- sinoatrial (SA) node in about 50% of people
- AV node in 90% of people.

The posterior descending artery supplies the posterior wall of the left ventricle in about 85% of people.

The left main coronary artery varies in length from a few millimeters to a few centimeters. It splits into two major branches, the left anterior descending (also known as the *interventricular*) and the left circumflex arteries. The left anterior descending artery runs down the anterior surface of the heart toward the apex. This artery and its branches—the diagonal arteries and the septal perforators—supply blood to the:

- anterior wall of the left ventricle
- anterior interventricular septum
- bundle of His
- right bundle branch
- anterior fasciculus of the left bundle branch.

The circumflex artery circles the left ventricle, ending on its posterior surface. The circumflex artery provides oxygenated blood to the:

- lateral wall of the left ventricle
- left atrium

- posterior wall of the left ventricle in 10% of people
- posterior fasciculus of the left bundle branch
- SA node in about 50% of people
- AV node in about 10% of people.

Collateral circulation

When two or more arteries supply the same region, they usually connect through anastomoses, junctions that provide alternate routes of blood flow. This network of smaller arteries, called *collateral circulation,* provides blood to capillaries that directly feed the heart muscle. Collateral circulation often becomes so strong that even if major coronary arteries become narrowed with plaque, collateral circulation can continue to supply blood to the heart.

Coronary artery blood flow

In contrast to the other vascular beds in the body, the heart receives its blood supply primarily during ventricular relaxation or diastole, when the left ventricle is filling with blood. This is because the coronary ostia lie near the aortic valve and become partially occluded when the aortic valve opens during ventricular contraction or systole. But when the aortic valve closes, the ostia are unobstructed, allowing blood to fill the coronary arteries. Because diastole is the time when the coronary arteries receive their blood supply, anything that shortens diastole, such as periods of increased heart rate or tachycardia, will also decrease coronary blood flow.

In addition, the left ventricular muscle compresses intramuscular vessels during systole. During diastole, the cardiac muscle relaxes and blood flow through the left ventricular capillaries is no longer obstructed.

Cardiac veins

Just like the other parts of the body, the heart has its own veins, which remove oxygen-depleted blood from the myocardium. About 75% of the total coronary venous blood flow leaves the left ventricle by way of the coronary sinus, an enlarged vessel that returns blood to the right atrium. Most of the venous blood from the right ventricle flows directly into the right atrium through the small anterior cardiac veins, not by way of the coronary sinus. A small amount of coronary blood flows back into the heart through the thebesian veins, tiny veins that empty directly into all chambers of the heart.

Cardiac physiology

This section addresses the heart's physiology, including the cardiac cycle, cardiac muscle innervation, depolarization and repolarization, and normal and abnormal impulse conduction.

THE CARDIAC CYCLE

The cardiac cycle comprises the events that occur from the beginning of one heartbeat to the beginning of the next. The cardiac cycle consists of ventricular diastole or relaxation and ventricular systole or contraction. During ventricular diastole, blood flows from the atria through the open tricuspid and mitral valves into the relaxed ventricles. The aortic and pulmonic valves close during ventricular diastole. (See *Phases of the cardiac cycle.*)

During diastole, about 75% of the blood flows passively from the atria through the open tricuspid and mitral valves and into the ventricles even before the atria contract. Atrial contraction, or atrial kick, contributes another 25% to ventricular filling. Loss of effective atrial contraction occurs in some arrhythmias, such as atrial fib-

Phases of the cardiac cycle

The cardiac cycle consists of five phases.

1. *Isovolumetric ventricular contraction.* In response to ventricular depolarization, tension in the ventricles increases. The rise in pressure within the ventricles causes the mitral and tricuspid valves to close. The pulmonic and aortic valves stay closed during the entire phase.

2. *Ventricular ejection.* When ventricular pressure exceeds aortic and pulmonary arterial pressure, the aortic and pulmonic valves open and the ventricles eject blood.

3. *Isovolumetric relaxation.* When ventricular pressure falls below pressure in the aorta and pulmonary artery, the aortic and pulmonic valves close. All valves are closed during this phase. Atrial diastole occurs as blood fills the atria.

4. *Ventricular filling.* Atrial pressure exceeds ventricular pressure, which causes the mitral and tricuspid valves to open. Blood then flows passively into the ventricles. About 70% of ventricular filling takes place during this phase.

5. *Atrial systole.* Known as the atrial kick, atrial systole (at the same time as late ventricular diastole) supplies the ventricles with the remaining 30% of the blood for each heartbeat.

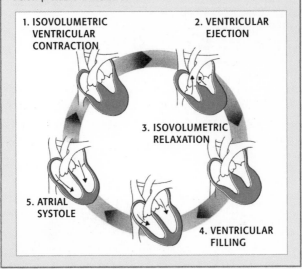

1. ISOVOLUMETRIC VENTRICULAR CONTRACTION

2. VENTRICULAR EJECTION

3. ISOVOLUMETRIC RELAXATION

4. VENTRICULAR FILLING

5. ATRIAL SYSTOLE

rillation, resulting in a subsequent reduction of cardiac output.

During ventricular systole, the mitral and tricuspid valves are closed as the relaxed atria fill with blood. As ventricular pressure rises, the aortic and pulmonic valves open. The ventricles contract and eject blood into the pulmonic and systemic circulation.

CARDIAC OUTPUT

Cardiac output is the amount of blood the left ventricle pumps into the aorta per minute. Cardiac output is measured by multiplying heart rate times stroke volume. Stroke volume is the amount of blood ejected with each ventricular contraction and is usually about 70 ml.

Normal cardiac output is 4 to 8 L/minute, depending on body size. The heart pumps only as much blood as the body requires, based on metabolic requirements. During exercise, for example, the heart increases cardiac output accordingly.

Three factors determine stroke volume:
■ preload
■ afterload
■ myocardial contractility. (See *Preload and afterload*.)

Preload

Preload is the degree of stretch or tension on the muscle fibers when they begin to contract. It's usually considered to be the end-diastolic pressure when the ventricle has filled.

Afterload

Afterload is the load or amount of pressure the left ventricle must work against to eject blood during systole and corresponds to the systolic pressure—the greater this re-

Preload and afterload

Preload refers to a passive stretching exerted by blood on the ventricular muscle fibers at the end of diastole. According to Starling's law, the more the cardiac muscles are stretched in diastole, the more forcefully they contract in systole, up to a certain point.

Afterload refers to the pressure that the ventricles need to generate to overcome higher pressure in the aorta to eject blood into the systemic circulation. This systemic vascular resistance corresponds to the systemic systolic pressure.

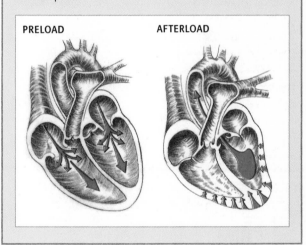

PRELOAD

AFTERLOAD

sistance, the greater the heart's workload. Afterload is also called the *systemic vascular resistance.*

Myocardial contractility

The degree of muscle fiber stretch at the end of diastole determines the ventricle's ability to contract, or contractility. The more the muscle fibers stretch during ventricular filling, up to an optimal length, the more forceful the contraction (Starling's law).

AUTONOMIC INNERVATION OF THE HEART

The two branches of the autonomic nervous system—the sympathetic (or adrenergic) and the parasympathetic (or cholinergic)—abundantly supply the heart. Sympathetic fibers innervate all the areas of the heart, while parasympathetic fibers primarily innervate the SA and AV nodes.

Sympathetic nerve stimulation causes the release of norepinephrine, which increases the heart rate by increasing SA-node discharge, accelerates AV node conduction time, and increases the force of myocardial contraction and cardiac output.

Parasympathetic (vagal) stimulation causes the release of acetylcholine, which produces the opposite effects. The rate of SA-node discharge is decreased, which results in a slow heart rate. AV node conduction time and cardiac output are also decreased.

ELECTRICAL IMPULSE TRANSMISSION

For the heart to contract and pump blood to the rest of the body, an electrical stimulus has to occur first. Generation and transmission of electrical impulses depend on the four key characteristics of cardiac cells:

- automaticity, which is a cell's ability to spontaneously create an electrical impulse (pacemaker cells usually possess this ability)
- excitability, which results from ion shifts across the cell membrane and refers to the cell's ability to respond to an electrical stimulus
- conductivity, which is the ability of a cell to transmit an electrical impulse from one cell to another
- contractility, which refers to the cell's ability to contract after receiving a stimulus by shortening and lengthening its muscle fibers.

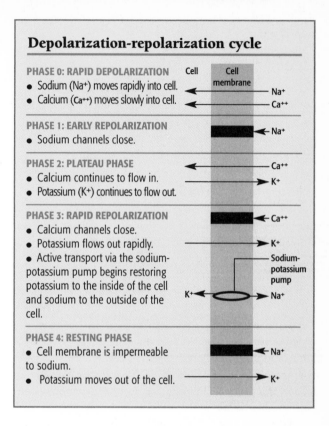

Depolarization-repolarization cycle

PHASE 0: RAPID DEPOLARIZATION
- Sodium (Na+) moves rapidly into cell.
- Calcium (Ca++) moves slowly into cell.

Cell   Cell membrane
← Na+
← Ca++

PHASE 1: EARLY REPOLARIZATION
- Sodium channels close.

← Na+

PHASE 2: PLATEAU PHASE
- Calcium continues to flow in.
- Potassium (K+) continues to flow out.

← Ca++
→ K+

PHASE 3: RAPID REPOLARIZATION
- Calcium channels close.
- Potassium flows out rapidly.
- Active transport via the sodium-potassium pump begins restoring potassium to the inside of the cell and sodium to the outside of the cell.

← Ca++
→ K+
Sodium-potassium pump
K+ ←   → Na+

PHASE 4: RESTING PHASE
- Cell membrane is impermeable to sodium.
- Potassium moves out of the cell.

← Na+
→ K+

It's important to remember that the first three characteristics are electrical properties of the cells and that the fourth characteristic, contractility, represents a mechanical response to the electrical activity. Of the four, automaticity has the greatest effect on cardiac rhythms.

DEPOLARIZATION AND REPOLARIZATION

As impulses are transmitted, cardiac cells undergo cycles of depolarization and repolarization. (See *Depolarization-repolarization cycle*, page 17.) Cardiac cells at rest are considered polarized, meaning that no electrical activity takes place. Cell membranes separate concentrations of ions, such as sodium and potassium, and create a more negative charge inside the cell. This is called the *resting potential*. After a stimulus occurs, ions cross the cell membrane and cause an action potential, or cell depolarization. When a cell is fully depolarized, it attempts to return to its resting state in a process called *repolarization*. Electrical charges in the cell reverse and return to normal.

Phases of depolarization-repolarization

A cycle of depolarization-repolarization consists of five phases—0 through 4. A curve that shows voltage changes during the five phases represents the action potential. (See *Action potential curves*.)

During phase 0 (rapid depolarization), the cell receives a stimulus, usually from a neighboring cell. The cell becomes more permeable to sodium, the inside of the cell becomes less negative, the cell is depolarized, and myocardial contraction occurs. In phase 1 (early repolarization), sodium stops flowing into the cell and the transmembrane potential falls slightly. Phase 2 (the plateau phase) is a prolonged period of slow repolarization, when little change occurs in the cell's transmembrane potential.

During phases 1 and 2 and at the beginning of phase 3, the cardiac cell is in its absolute refractory period. During that period, no stimulus, no matter how strong, can excite the cell.

Phase 3 (rapid repolarization) occurs as the cell returns to its original state. During the last half of this phase, when the cell in its relatively refractory period, a very strong stimulus can depolarize it.

Phase 4 is the resting phase of the action potential. By the end of phase 4, the cell is ready for another stimulus.

Action potential curves

An action potential curve shows the changes in a cell's electrical charge during the five phases of the depolarization-repolarization cycle. These graphs show electrical changes for pacemaker and nonpacemaker cells.

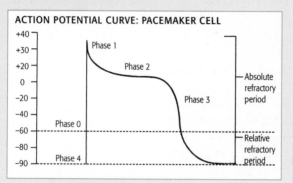

As the graph below shows, the action potential curve for pacemaker cells, such as those in the sinoatrial node, differs from that of other myocardial cells. Pacemaker cells have a resting membrane potential of –60 millivolts (mV), instead of –90 mV, and begin to depolarize spontaneously. Called *diastolic depolarization,* this effect results primarily from calcium and sodium leaking into the cell.

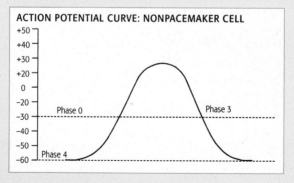

An ECG shows the electrical activity of the heart. Keep in mind that the ECG represents electrical activity only, not the mechanical activity or actual pumping of the heart.

CONDUCTION SYSTEM OF THE HEART

After depolarization and repolarization occur, the resulting electrical impulse travels through the heart along a pathway called the *conduction system*. (See *Cardiac conduction system*.)

Impulses travel from the SA node through the internodal tracts and Bachmann's bundle to the AV node. From there, impulses travel through the bundle of His and the bundle branches to the Purkinje fibers.

SA node

The SA node, located in the right atrium where the superior vena cava joins the atrial tissue mass, is the heart's main pacemaker. Under resting conditions, the SA node generates 60 to 100 impulses/minute. When initiated, the impulses follow a specific path through the heart. They usually don't travel in a backward or retrograde direction because the cells can't respond to a stimulus immediately after depolarizing.

From the SA node, impulses travel through the right and left atria. In the right atrium, impulses are believed to be transmitted along three internodal tracts, sometimes referred to as the *interatrial tracts*. They are the anterior, middle (Wenckebach's), and posterior (Thorel's) internodal tracts.

The impulses travel through the left atrium via Bachmann's bundle, tracts of tissue extending from the SA node to the left atrium. Impulse transmission through the right and left atria occurs so rapidly that the atria contract almost simultaneously.

Cardiac conduction system

Specialized fibers transmit electrical impulses throughout the heart's cell, causing the heart to contract. This illustration shows the elements of the cardiac conduction system.

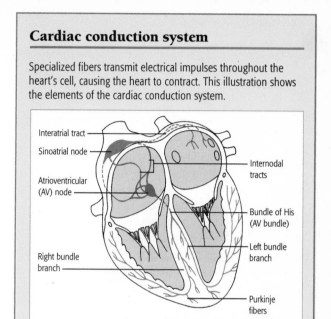

AV node

The AV node is in the inferior right atrium near the ostium of the coronary sinus. Although the AV node doesn't have pacemaker cells, the tissue surrounding it, referred to as *junctional tissue,* has pacemaker cells that can fire at a rate of 40 to 60 beats/minute. As the AV node conducts the atrial impulse to the ventricles, it causes a 0.04-second delay. This delay allows the ventricles to complete their filling phase as the atria contract. It also allows the cardiac muscle to stretch to its fullest for peak cardiac output.

Bundle of His and bundle branches

Rapid conduction then resumes through the bundle of His, which divides into the right and left bundle branches. The branches extend down both sides of the interventricular septum:

■ The right bundle branch extends down the right side of the interventricular septum and through the right ventricle.

■ The left bundle branch extends down the left side of the interventricular septum and through the left ventricle.

As a pacemaker site, the bundle of His has a firing rate of 40 to 60 beats/minute. The bundle of His usually fires when the SA node fails to generate an impulse at a normal rate or when the impulse fails to reach the AV junction.

The left bundle branch then splits into two branches, or fasciculations:

■ The left anterior fasciculus extends through the anterior portion of the left ventricle.

■ The left posterior fasciculus extends through the lateral and posterior portions of the left ventricle.

Impulses travel much faster down the left bundle branch, which feeds the larger, thicker-walled left ventricle, than down the right bundle branch, which feeds the smaller, thinner-walled right ventricle. The difference in the conduction speed allows both ventricles to contract at the same time. The entire network of specialized nervous tissue that extends through the ventricles is called the *His-Purkinje system*.

Purkinje system

Purkinje fibers are part of a diffuse muscle fiber network under the endocardium that transmits impulses quicker than any other part of the conduction system. This pacemaker site usually doesn't fire unless the SA and AV nodes fail to generate an impulse or when the normal impulse is blocked in both bundle branches. The automatic firing rate of the Purkinje fibers ranges from 15 to 40 beats/minute.

LIFE STAGES In children younger than age 3, the AV node may discharge impulses at a rate of 50 to 80 times per minute; the Purkinje fibers may discharge at a rate of 40 to 50 times per minute.

ABNORMAL IMPULSE CONDUCTION

Causes of abnormal impulse conduction include altered automaticity, retrograde conduction of impulses, reentry abnormalities, and ectopy.

Altered automaticity

Automaticity, a special characteristic of pacemaker cells, allows them to generate electrical impulses spontaneously. If a cell's automaticity increases or decreases, an arrhythmia—or abnormality in the cardiac rhythm—can occur. Tachycardia and premature beats are commonly caused by an increase in the automaticity of pacemaker cells below the SA node. Likewise, a decrease in automaticity of cells in the SA node can cause the development of bradycardia or escape rhythms generated by lower pacemaker sites.

Retrograde conduction

Impulses that begin below the AV node can be transmitted back toward the atria. This backward, or retrograde, conduction usually takes longer than normal conduction and can cause the atria and ventricles to lose synchrony.

Reentry

Reentry occurs when the same impulse activates cardiac tissue two or more times. This may happen when conduction speed slows or when the refractory periods for neighboring cells occur at different times. Impulses are delayed long enough that cells have time to repolarize. In those cases, the active impulse reenters the same area and produces another impulse.

Ectopy

Injured pacemaker (or nonpacemaker) cells may partially depolarize, rather than fully depolarizing. Partial depolarization can lead to spontaneous or secondary depolarization, repetitive ectopic firings called *triggered activity*.

2

BASIC ELECTROCARDIOGRAPHY

One of the most valuable diagnostic tools available, an electrocardiogram (ECG) records the heart's electrical activity as waveforms. By interpreting these waveforms accurately, you can identify rhythm disturbances, conduction abnormalities, and electrolyte imbalances. An ECG aids in diagnosing and monitoring conditions, such as myocardial infarction (MI) and pericarditis.

To interpret an ECG correctly, you must:
- recognize its key components
- analyze them separately
- put your findings together to reach a conclusion about the heart's electrical activity.

This chapter will explain that analysis, beginning with some fundamental information about electrocardiography.

How an electrocardiograph works

The heart's electrical activity produces currents that radiate through the surrounding tissue to the skin. When electrodes are attached to the skin, they sense those currents and transmit them to the electrocardiograph. The electrocardiograph transforms this electrical activity into waveforms that represent the heart's depolarization-repolarization cycle.

Myocardial depolarization occurs when a wave of stimulation passes through the heart and causes the heart muscle to contract. Repolarization is the relaxation phase. An ECG shows the precise sequence of electrical events that happen in the cardiac cells throughout that process and identifies rhythm disturbances and conduction abnormalities.

Leads and planes

Because the electrical currents from the heart radiate to the skin in many directions, electrodes are placed at different locations to get a total picture of the heart's electrical activity. The electrocardiograph can then record information from different perspectives, which are called *leads* and *planes*.

LEADS

A lead provides a view of the heart's electrical activity between two points, or poles. Each lead consists of one positive and one negative pole. Between the two poles lies an imaginary line representing the lead's *axis,* a term that refers to the direction of the current moving through the heart. Because each lead measures the heart's electrical potential from different directions, each generates its own characteristic tracing. (See *Current direction and waveform deflection.*)

These tracings all look different, so understanding what's considered normal for each lead helps to interpret rhythms. (See *Looking at the 12 leads of the same rhythm,* page 28.)

Waveform appearance

The direction in which the electrical current flows determines how the waveforms appear on the ECG tracing.

Current direction and waveform deflection

This illustration shows possible directions of electrical current and the corresponding waveform deflections. The direction of the electrical current determines the upward or downward deflection of an electrocardiogram waveform.

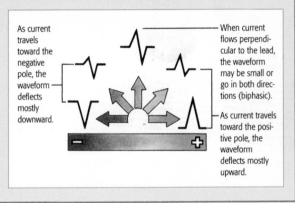

As current travels toward the negative pole, the waveform deflects mostly downward.

When current flows perpendicular to the lead, the waveform may be small or go in both directions (biphasic).

As current travels toward the positive pole, the waveform deflects mostly upward.

When the current flows along the axis toward the positive pole of the electrode, the waveform deflects upward and is called a *positive deflection*. When the current flows away from the positive pole, the waveform deflects downward, below the baseline, and is called *a negative deflection*. When the current flows perpendicular to the axis, the wave may go in both directions (biphasic) or be unusually small. When electrical activity is absent or too small to measure, the waveform is a straight line, also called an *isoelectric deflection*.

PLANES

A plane is a cross section of the heart, which provides a different view of the heart's electrical activity. In the frontal

Looking at the 12 leads of the same rhythm

These 12 tracings are from the 12 leads of a 12-lead electrocardiogram. They're all of the same heart rhythm. The flow of current, either to or away from the positive pole, results in positive and negative deflections.

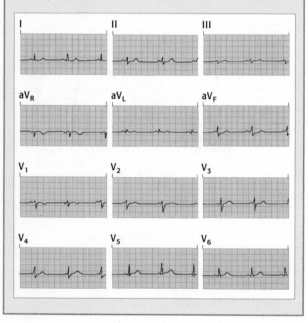

plane—a vertical cut through the middle of the heart from top to bottom—electrical activity is viewed from an anterior to posterior approach. The six limb leads of a 12-lead ECG are viewed from the frontal plane.

In the horizontal plane—a transverse cut through the middle of the heart, dividing it into upper and lower portions—electrical activity can be viewed from a superior or an inferior approach. The six chest, or precordial, leads of a 12-lead ECG are viewed from the horizontal plane.

Types of ECG recordings

The two main types of ECG recordings are the 12-lead ECG and a rhythm strip, which may record one or more selected leads. Both types give valuable information about the heart's electrical activity.

12-LEAD ECG
A 12-lead ECG records information from 12 different views of the heart and provides a complete picture of electrical activity. These 12 views are obtained by placing electrodes on the patient's limbs and chest. The limb leads and the precordial leads reflect information from the different planes of the heart.

Limb leads
Different leads provide different information. The six limb leads that provide information about the heart's frontal plane are:
■ leads I, II, and III, which require a negative and positive electrode, making them bipolar
■ augmented vector right (aV_R), augmented vector left (aV_L), and augmented vector foot (aV_F), which require only a positive electrode, making them unipolar.

Chest leads
The six precordial or V leads — V_1, V_2, V_3, V_4, V_5, and V_6 — provide information about the heart's horizontal plane. Like the augmented leads, the precordial leads are unipolar, requiring only a positive electrode. The electrocardiograph calculates the negative pole of these leads, which is in the center of the heart.

RHYTHM STRIP

A rhythm strip provides information about the heart's electrical activity from one or more leads simultaneously and can be used to monitor cardiac status. Chest electrodes pick up the heart's electrical activity for display on the monitor. The monitor also displays heart rate and other measurements and prints out strips of cardiac rhythms. Commonly monitored leads include leads I, II, and III and V_1 and V_6.

ECG MONITORING SYSTEMS

The type of ECG monitoring system used—hardwire monitoring or telemetry—depends on what's available in the facility and is commonly guided by the patient's condition.

HARDWIRE MONITORING

With hardwire monitoring, the electrodes on the patient's chest connect to a leadwire cable that connects directly to the bedside cardiac monitor. Most hardwire monitors are mounted permanently on a shelf or wall near the patient's bed. Some monitors are mounted on an I.V. pole for portability and have defibrillating and transcutaneous pacing capability.

The cardiac monitor:
■ provides a continuous cardiac rhythm display
■ transmits the ECG tracing to a console at the nurses' station.

Both the monitor and the console have alarms that sound when the heart rate falls below or exceeds set limits or when arrhythmias occur. Both can also print rhythm strips. Hardwire monitors usually have the ability to track:
■ pulse oximetry
■ blood pressure
■ hemodynamic measurements

■ other parameters through various attachments to the
patient.

Intensive care units and emergency departments generally use hardwire monitoring because it permits continuous observation of one or more patients from more than
one area in the unit. However, this type of monitoring
does have disadvantages, including limited mobility because the patient is connected to the monitor.

TELEMETRY MONITORING

With telemetry monitoring, the electrodes on the patient's
chest connect to a leadwire cable that connects to a small,
battery-powered transmitter carried in a pocket or pouch
that sends electrical signals to a central station, where the
signals are displayed on a monitor screen. This type of
ECG monitoring allows the patient more freedom in his
activities.

Electrode placement

Different leads provide different views of the heart. A lead
may be chosen to highlight a particular part of the ECG
complex or the electrical events of a specific area of the
heart.

Although leads II, V_1, and V_6 are among the most
commonly used leads for continuous monitoring, lead se-
lection varies by the patient's condition. If your monitoring system has the capability, you may also monitor the
patient in more than one lead. (See *Dual lead monitoring*,
page 32.)

STANDARD LIMB LEADS

All standard limb leads or bipolar limb leads have a third
electrode, known as the *ground*, which is placed on the
chest to prevent electrical interference from appearing on

Dual lead monitoring

Monitoring in two leads provides a more complete picture than monitoring in one. With simultaneous dual monitoring, you'll generally review the first lead—usually designated as the primary lead—for arrhythmias.

A two-lead view helps detect ectopic beats or aberrant rhythms.

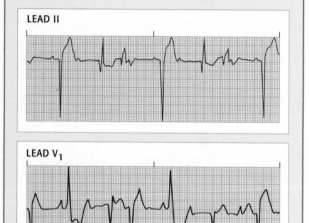

LEAD II

LEAD V₁

the ECG recording. The axes of the three bipolar limb leads — I, II, and III — form a triangle around the heart and provide a frontal plane view of the heart. (See *Einthoven's triangle*.)

Lead I

Lead I provides a view of the heart that shows current moving from right to left. Because current flows from neg-

Einthoven's triangle

The axes of the three bipolar limb leads (I, II, and III) form a triangle, known as *Einthoven's triangle*. Because the electrodes for these leads are about equidistant from the heart, the triangle is equilateral.

The axis of lead I extends from shoulder to shoulder, with the right arm lead being the negative electrode and the left arm lead being the positive electrode. The axis of lead II runs from the negative right arm lead electrode to the positive left leg lead electrode. The axis of lead III extends from the negative left arm lead electrode to the positive left leg lead electrode.

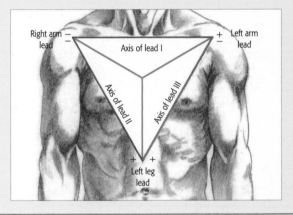

ative to positive, the positive electrode for this lead is placed on the left arm or on the left side of the chest, just below the clavicle; the negative electrode is placed on the right arm or on the right side of the chest, just below the clavicle. Lead I produces a positive deflection on ECG tracings and is helpful in monitoring atrial rhythms and hemiblocks.

Lead II

In lead II, the positive electrode is placed on the patient's left leg; the negative electrode, on the right arm. For continuous monitoring, the electrodes are placed on the torso for convenience, with the positive electrode below the lowest palpable rib at the left midclavicular line and the negative electrode below the right clavicle. The current travels down and to the left in this lead. Lead II tends to produce a positive, high-voltage deflection, resulting in tall P, R, and T waves. This lead is useful for detecting sinus node and atrial arrhythmias.

Lead III

Lead III usually produces a positive deflection. The positive electrode is placed on the left leg; the negative electrode, on the left arm. For continuous monitoring, the electrodes are placed on the chest, with the positive electrode below the lowest palpable rib at the left midclavicular line and the negative electrode below the left clavicle. Along with lead II, this lead is useful for detecting changes in an inferior-wall MI.

AUGMENTED UNIPOLAR LEADS

Leads aV_R, aV_L, and aV_F are called *augmented leads* because the small waveforms that normally would appear from these unipolar leads are enhanced by the ECG.

In lead aV_R, the positive electrode is placed on the right arm and produces a negative deflection because the heart's electrical activity moves away from the lead. In lead aV_L, the positive electrode is placed on the left arm and usually produces a positive deflection on the ECG. In lead aV_F, the positive electrode is placed on the left leg (despite the name aV_F) and produces a positive deflection. These three limb leads also provide a view of the heart's frontal plane.

Precordial views

These illustrations show the different views of the heart obtained from each precordial (chest) lead.

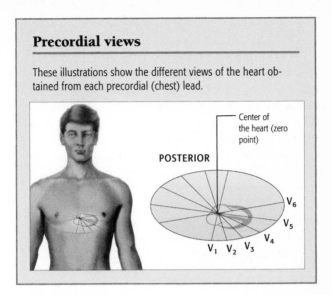

PRECORDIAL UNIPOLAR LEADS

The six unipolar precordial leads are placed in sequence across the chest and provide a view of the heart's horizontal plane. (See *Precordial views.*)

The precordial lead V_1 electrode is placed on the right side of the sternum at the fourth intercostal space. This lead shows the P wave, QRS complex, and ST segment particularly well. It helps to distinguish between right and left ventricular ectopic beats that result from myocardial irritation or other cardiac stimulation outside the normal conduction system. Lead V_1 is also useful in monitoring ventricular arrhythmias, ST-segment changes, and bundle-branch blocks.

Lead V_2 is placed to the left of the sternum at the fourth intercostal space.

Lead V_3 goes between V_2 and V_4 at the fifth inter-costal space. Leads V_1, V_2, and V_3 are biphasic, with positive and negative deflections. Leads V_2 and V_3 can be used to detect ST-segment elevation.

Lead V_4 is placed at the fifth intercostal space at the midclavicular line and produces a biphasic waveform.

Lead V_5 is placed at the fifth intercostal space at the anterior axillary line. Lead V_5 produces a positive deflection on the ECG and, along with V_4, can show changes in the ST segment or T wave.

Lead V_6, the last of the precordial leads, is placed level with lead V4 at the midaxillary line. Lead V_6 produces a positive deflection on the ECG. Precordial lead electrodes (V_1 through V_6) must be placed in the same place consistently. Any variation, even as small as 1 centimeter, may alter waveforms. Serial 12-lead ECGs and consistent ST-segment monitoring depend on consistent lead placement.

MODIFIED CHEST LEADS

MCL_1 is similar to lead V_1 on the 12-lead ECG and is created by placing the negative electrode on the left upper chest below the clavicle, the positive electrode on the right side of the heart in the fourth intercostal space, and the ground electrode usually on the right upper chest below the clavicle.

When the positive electrode is on the right side of the heart and the electrical current travels toward the left ventricle, the waveform has a negative deflection. As a result, ectopic or abnormal beats deflect in a positive direction.

You can use this lead to:

■ monitor premature ventricular beats
■ distinguish different types of tachycardia, such as ventricular and supraventricular tachycardia
■ assess bundle-branch defects and P-wave changes
■ confirm pacemaker wire placement.

MCL$_6$ may be used as an alternative to MCL$_1$. Like MCL$_1$, it monitors ventricular conduction changes. The positive lead in MCL$_6$ is placed in the same location as its equivalent, lead V$_6$, for which the positive electrode is placed in the left fifth intercostal space at the midaxillary line, the negative electrode below the left shoulder, and the ground below the right shoulder.

Leadwire systems

A three- or five-electrode leadwire system may be used for cardiac monitoring. (See *Leadwire systems,* pages 38 and 39.) Both systems use a ground electrode to prevent accidentally giving the patient an electrical shock.

A three-electrode system has one positive electrode, one negative electrode, and a ground. The five-electrode system has a right leg electrode that becomes a permanent ground for all leads and uses an additional exploratory chest lead to allow you to monitor any six chest leads as well as the standard limb leads. (See *Using a five-leadwire system,* page 40.) This system uses standardized chest placement. Wires that attach to the electrodes are usually color-coded to help you place them correctly on the patient's chest.

Application of electrodes

Before attaching electrodes to your patient, make sure he knows you're monitoring his heart rate and rhythm, not controlling them. Tell him not to become upset if he hears an alarm during the procedure; it probably just means a leadwire has come loose.

Explain the electrode placement procedure to the patient, provide privacy, and wash your hands. Expose the

Leadwire systems

This chart shows the correct electrode positions for some of the leads you'll use most often–the five-leadwire, three-leadwire, and telemetry systems. The chart uses the abbreviations RA for the right arm, LA for the left arm, RL for the right leg, LL for the left leg, C for the chest, and G for the ground.

ELECTRODE POSITIONS
In the three- and five-leadwire systems, electrode positions for one lead may be identical to those for another lead. When that happens, change the lead selector switch to the setting that corresponds to the lead you want. In some cases, you'll need to reposition the electrodes.

TELEMETRY
In a telemetry monitoring system, you can create the same leads as the other systems with just two electrodes and a ground wire.

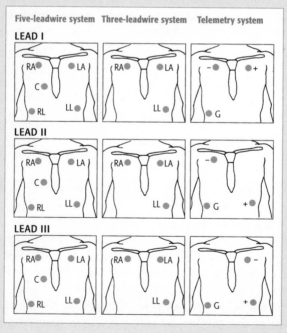

Five-leadwire system   Three-leadwire system   Telemetry system

LEAD I

LEAD II

LEAD III

Leadwire systems *(continued)*

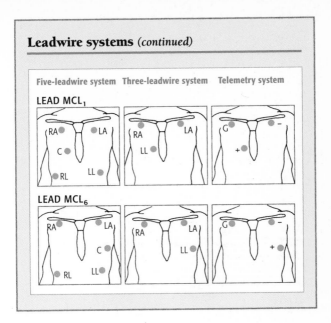

Five-leadwire system   Three-leadwire system   Telemetry system

LEAD MCL₁

LEAD MCL₆

patient's chest, and select electrode sites for the chosen lead. Choose sites over soft tissues or close to bone, not over bony prominences, thick muscles, or skin folds. Those areas can produce ECG artifacts—waveforms not produced by the heart's electrical activity.

SKIN PREPARATION

Next, prepare the patient's skin. Wash the chest with soap and water, and dry it thoroughly. Hair may interfere with electrical contact; therefore, it may be necessary to clip dense hair with clippers or scissors. Then use a special rough patch on the back of the electrode, a dry washcloth, or a gauze pad to briskly rub each site until the skin reddens. Be careful not to damage or break the skin. Brisk scrubbing helps to remove dead skin cells and improves electrical contact. If the patient has oily skin, clean each

Using a five-leadwire system

This illustration shows the correct placement of the electrodes for a five-leadwire system. The chest electrode shown is located in the lead V_1 position, but you can place it in any of the chest-lead positions. The leadwires that attach to the electrodes are color-coded as follows.

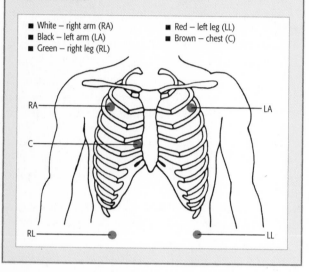

- White – right arm (RA)
- Black – left arm (LA)
- Green – right leg (RL)

- Red – left leg (LL)
- Brown – chest (C)

site with an alcohol pad and let it air-dry. This ensures proper adhesion and prevents alcohol from becoming trapped beneath the electrode, which can irritate the skin and cause skin breakdown.

APPLICATION OF ELECTRODE PADS

To apply the electrodes, remove the backing and make sure each pregelled electrode is still moist. If an electrode has become dry, discard it and select another. A dry electrode decreases electrical contact and interferes with waveforms.

Apply one electrode to each prepared site using this method:

■ Press one side of the electrode against the patient's skin, pull gently, and then press the opposite side of the electrode against the skin.

■ Using two fingers, press the adhesive edge around the outside of the electrode to the patient's chest. This fixes the gel and stabilizes the electrode.

■ Repeat this procedure for each electrode.

■ Every 24 hours, remove the electrodes, assess the patient's skin, and replace the old electrodes with new ones.

ATTACHING LEADWIRES

You'll also need to attach leadwires to the monitor by a cable connection. Then attach leadwires to the electrodes. Leadwires may clip on or, more commonly, snap on. If you're using the snap-on type, attach the electrode to the leadwire immediately before applying it to the patient's chest. This will help to prevent patient discomfort and disturbances of the contact between the electrode and the skin. When you use a clip-on leadwire, apply it after the electrode has been secured to the patient's skin. That way, applying the clip won't interfere with the electrode's contact with the skin.

Observing cardiac rhythm

After the electrodes are in proper position, the monitor is on, and the necessary cables are attached, observe the screen. You should see the patient's ECG waveform. Although some monitoring systems allow you to make adjustments by touching the screen, most require you to manipulate knobs and buttons. If the waveform appears too large or too small, change the size by adjusting the gain control. If the waveform appears too high or too low on the screen, adjust the position dial.

Verify that the monitor detects each heartbeat by comparing the patient's apical rate with the rate displayed on the monitor. Set the upper and lower limits of the heart rate according to your facility's policy and the patient's condition. Heart rate alarms are generally set 10 to 20 beats per minute higher or lower than the patient's heart rate.

OBTAINING AND DOCUMENTING HEART RHYTHMS

Monitors with arrhythmia detection generate a rhythm strip automatically whenever the alarm goes off. You can obtain other views of your patient's cardiac rhythm by selecting different leads. You can select leads with the lead-selector button or switch.

To get a printout of the patient's cardiac rhythm, press the record control on the monitor. The ECG strip will be printed at the central console. Some systems print the rhythm from a recorder box on the monitor itself.

Most monitors print the patient's name, room number, date, time, and interpretation on the recording, but if the monitor you're using doesn't do this, label the rhythm strip with the patient's name, room number, date, time, and rhythm interpretation. Add other information, such as:

■ drugs given
■ presence of chest pain
■ patient activity at the time of the recording.

Make sure you place the rhythm strip in the appropriate section of the patient's medical record.

ECG grid

This electrocardiogram (ECG) grid shows the horizontal axis and vertical axis and their respective measurement values.

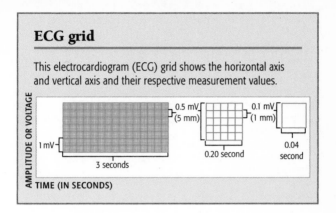

ECG RECORDING PAPER

Waveforms produced by the heart's electrical current are recorded on graphed ECG paper by a stylus. ECG paper consists of horizontal and vertical lines forming a grid. The piece of paper that the ECG appears on is called an *ECG strip* or *tracing*. (See *ECG grid*.)

Horizontal axis

The horizontal axis of the ECG strip represents time. Each small block equals 0.04 second; five small blocks form a large block, which equals 0.20 second. Determine this time increment by multiplying 0.04 second (for one small block) by 5, the number of small blocks that compose a large block. Five large blocks equal 1 second (5 × 0.20). When measuring or calculating a patient's heart rate, use a 6-second strip consisting of 30 large blocks.

Vertical axis

The ECG strip's vertical axis measures amplitude in millimeters (mm) or voltage in millivolts (mV). Each small block represents 1 mm or 0.1 mV; each large block, 5 mm or 0.5 mV. To determine the amplitude of a wave, segment, or interval, count the number of small blocks from the baseline to the highest or lowest point of the wave, segment, or interval.

Troubleshooting monitor problems

For optimal cardiac monitoring, you need to recognize problems that can interfere with obtaining a reliable ECG recording. (See *The look of monitor problems.*) Causes of interference include artifacts from patient movement and poorly placed or poorly functioning equipment.

ARTIFACTS

Artifacts, also called *waveform interference,* may be seen with excessive movement (somatic tremor). The baseline of the ECG appears wavy, bumpy, or tremulous. Dry electrodes may also cause this problem due to poor contact.

Artifacts may also be caused by electrical interference or AC interference (60-cycle interference). This may be due to interference from other room equipment or improperly grounded equipment. As a result, the lost current pulses at a rate of 60 cycles per second. This interference appears on the ECG as a baseline that's thick and unreadable. Faulty equipment, such as broken leadwires and cables, can also cause monitoring problems.

Some types of artifacts resemble arrhythmias, and the monitor will interpret them as such. For example, the monitor may sense a small movement, such as the patient brushing his teeth, as a lethal ventricular tachycardia. Remember to always treat the patient, not the monitor. The more familiar you become with your unit's monitoring system—and with your patient—the more quickly you can recognize and interpret problems and act appropriately.

The look of monitor problems

This chart illustrates the most commonly encountered monitor problems and explains how to identify them, possible causes, and recommended interventions.

WAVEFORM	POSSIBLE CAUSE	INTERVENTIONS
ARTIFACT (WAVEFORM INTERFERENCE) 	• Patient experiencing seizures, chills, or anxiety	• If the patient is having a seizure, notify the practitioner and intervene as ordered. • Keep the patient warm, and encourage him to relax.
	• Dirty or corroded connections • Improper electrode application	• Replace dirty or corroded wires. • Check the electrodes and reapply them if needed. Clean the patient's skin well because skin oils and dead skin cells inhibit conduction. • Check the electrode gel. If the gel is dry, apply new electrodes.
	• Short circuit in leadwires or cable	• Replace broken equipment.
	• Electrical interference from other equipment in the room	• Make sure all electrical equipment is attached to a common ground. Check all three-pronged plugs to ensure that none of the prongs is loose. Notify biomedical department.
	• Static electricity interference from inadequate room humidity	• Regulate room humidity to 40%, if possible.
FALSE-HIGH-RATE ALARM	• Gain setting too high, particularly with MCL_1 setting	• Assess the patient for signs and symptoms of hyperkalemia. • Reset gain.
	• HIGH alarm set too low, or LOW alarm set too high	• Set alarm limits according to the patient's heart rate.

(continued)

The look of monitor problems (*continued*)

WAVEFORM	POSSIBLE CAUSE	INTERVENTIONS
WEAK SIGNALS	● Improper electrode application	● Reapply the electrodes.
	● QRS complex too small to register	● Reset gain so that the height of the complex is greater than 1 mV. ● Try monitoring the patient on another lead.
	● Wire or cable failure	● Replace faulty wires or cables.
WANDERING BASELINE	● Patient restless	● Encourage the patient to relax.
	● Chest wall movement during respiration	● Make sure that tension on the cable isn't pulling the electrode away from the patient's body.
	● Improper electrode application; electrode positioned over bone	● Reposition improperly placed electrodes.
FUZZY BASELINE (ELECTRICAL INTERFERENCE)	● Electrical interference from other equipment in the room	● Make sure that all electrical equipment is attached to a common ground. ● Check all three-pronged plugs to make sure none of the prongs are loose.
	● Improper grounding of the patient's bed	● Make sure that the bed ground is attached to the room's common ground.
	● Electrode malfunction	● Replace the electrodes.

The look of monitor problems *(continued)*

WAVEFORM	POSSIBLE CAUSE	INTERVENTIONS
BASELINE (NO WAVEFORM)	● Improper electrode placement (perpendicular to axis of heart)	● Reposition improperly placed electrodes.
	● Electrode disconnected ● Dry electrode gel	● Check whether electrodes are disconnected. ● Check electrode gel. If the gel is dry, apply new electrodes.
	● Wire or cable failure	● Replace faulty wires or cables.

WANDERING BASELINE

A wandering baseline undulates, meaning that all waveforms are present but the baseline isn't stationary. Movement of the chest wall during respiration, poor electrode placement, or poor electrode contact usually causes this problem.

Analyzing a rhythm strip

An ECG complex represents the electrical events that occur during one cardiac cycle. A complex consists of five waveforms labeled with the letters P, Q, R, S, and T. The middle three letters—Q, R, and S—are referred to as a unit, the QRS complex. ECG tracings represent the conduction of electrical impulses from the atria to the ventricles. (See *ECG waveform components,* page 48.)

ECG waveform components

This illustration shows the components of a normal ECG waveform.

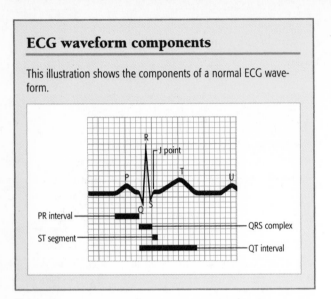

P WAVE

The P wave is the first component of a normal ECG waveform. It represents atrial depolarization or conduction of an electrical impulse through the atria. When evaluating a P wave, look closely at its characteristics, especially its location, configuration, and deflection. A normal P wave has these characteristics:

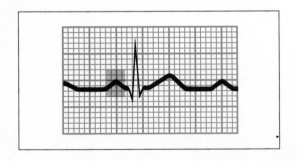

- location: precedes the QRS complex
- amplitude: 2 to 3 mm high
- duration: 0.06 to 0.12 second
- configuration: usually rounded and upright
- deflection: positive or upright in leads I, II, aV_F, and V_2 to V_6; usually positive but may vary in leads III and aV_L; negative or inverted in lead aV_R; biphasic or variable in lead V_1.

If the deflection and configuration of a P wave are normal—for example, if the P wave is upright in lead II and is rounded and smooth—and if the P wave precedes each QRS complex, you can assume that this electrical impulse originated in the sinoatrial (SA) node. The atria start to contract partway through the P wave, but you won't see this on the ECG. Remember, the ECG records electrical activity only, not mechanical activity or contraction.

P-wave variations

Peaked, notched, or enlarged P waves may represent atrial hypertrophy or enlargement associated with chronic obstructive pulmonary disease, pulmonary emboli, valvular disease, or heart failure. Inverted P waves may signify retrograde or reverse conduction from the atrioventricular (AV) junction toward the atria. Whenever an upright sinus P wave becomes inverted, consider retrograde or reverse conduction as a possible condition. (See *Different P-wave configurations,* page 50.)

Varying P waves indicate that the impulse may be coming from different sites, as with a wandering pacemaker rhythm, irritable atrial tissue, or damage near the SA node. Absent P waves may signify conduction by a route other than the SA node, as with a junctional or atrial fibrillation rhythm. When a P wave doesn't precede the QRS complex, complete heart block may be present.

Different P-wave configurations

A P wave may be configured on lead II in the following ways:

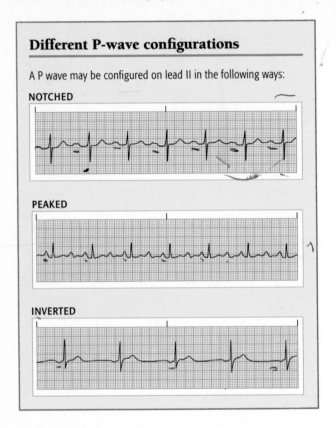

NOTCHED

PEAKED

INVERTED

PR INTERVAL

The PR interval tracks the atrial impulse from the atria through the AV node, bundle of His, and right and left bundle branches. When evaluating a PR interval, look especially at its duration. Changes in the PR interval indicate an altered impulse formation or a conduction delay, as seen in AV block. A normal PR interval has these characteristics (amplitude, configuration, and deflection aren't measured):

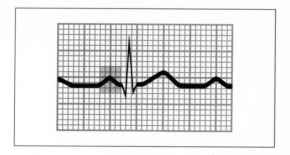

■ location: from the beginning of the P wave to the beginning of the QRS complex

■ duration: 0.12 to 0.20 second.

These characteristics are different for pediatric patients. (See *Pediatric rates and intervals,* page 52.)

PR interval abnormalities

Short PR intervals (less than 0.12 second) indicate that the impulse originated somewhere other than the SA node. This variation is associated with junctional arrhythmias and preexcitation syndromes. Prolonged PR intervals (greater than 0.20 second) may represent a conduction delay through the atria or AV junction due to digoxin toxicity or heart block—slowing related to ischemia or conduction tissue disease.

QRS COMPLEX

The QRS complex follows the P wave and represents depolarization of the ventricles, or impulse conduction. Immediately after the ventricles depolarize, as represented by the QRS complex, they contract. That contraction:

■ ejects blood from the ventricles

■ pumps it through the arteries

■ creates a pulse.

LIFE STAGES

Pediatric rates and intervals

The hearts of infants and children beat faster than those of adults because children have smaller ventricular size and higher metabolic needs. The fast heart rate and small size produces short PR intervals and QRS intervals.

AGE	HEART RATE (beats/minute)	PR INTERVAL (in seconds)	QRS INTERVAL (in seconds)
1 to 3 weeks	100 to 180	0.07 to 0.14	0.03 to 0.07
1 to 6 months	100 to 185	0.07 to 0.16	0.03 to 0.07
7 to 11 months	100 to 170	0.08 to 0.16	0.03 to 0.08
1 to 3 years	90 to 150	0.09 to 0.16	0.03 to 0.08
4 to 5 years	70 to 140	0.09 to 0.16	0.03 to 0.08
5 to 7 years	65 to 130	0.09 to 0.16	0.03 to 0.08
8 to 11 years	60 to 110	0.09 to 0.16	0.03 to 0.09
12 to 16 years	60 to 100	0.09 to 0.18	0.03 to 0.09

Whenever you're monitoring cardiac rhythm, remember that the waveform you see represents the heart's electrical activity only. It doesn't guarantee a mechanical contraction of the heart and a subsequent pulse. The contraction could be weak, as happens with premature ventricular contractions, or absent, as happens with pulseless electrical activity. So before you treat the strip, check the patient.

Pay special attention to the duration and configuration when evaluating a QRS complex. A normal complex has these characteristics:

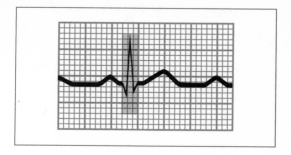

- location: follows the PR interval
- amplitude: 5 to 30 mm high but differs for each lead used
- duration: 0.06 to 0.10 second, or half of the PR interval (Measure duration from the beginning of the Q wave to the end of the S wave or from the beginning of the R wave if the Q wave is absent.)
- configuration: consists of the Q wave (the first negative deflection, or deflection below the baseline, after the P wave), the R wave (the first positive deflection after the Q wave), and the S wave (the first negative deflection after the R wave). You may not always see all three waves. The ventricles depolarize quickly, minimizing contact time between the stylus and the ECG paper, so the QRS complex typically appears thinner than other ECG components. It may also look different in each lead. (See *QRS waveform variety,* page 54.)
- deflection: positive (with most of the complex above the baseline) in leads I, II, III, aV_L, aV_F, and V_4 to V_6 and negative in leads aV_R and V_1 to V_3.

QRS wave variations

Remember that the QRS complex represents intraventricular conduction time. That's why identifying and correctly interpreting it is so crucial. If no P wave appears with the

QRS waveform variety

These illustrations show the various configurations of QRS complexes. When documenting the QRS complex, use upper-case letters to indicate a wave with a normal or high amplitude (greater than 5 mm) and lowercase letters to indicate one with a low amplitude (less than 5 mm).

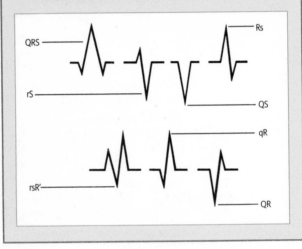

QRS complex, then the impulse may have originated in the ventricles, indicating a ventricular arrhythmia.

Deep, wide Q waves may represent MI. In this case, the Q-wave amplitude (depth) is greater than or equal to 25% of the height of the succeeding R wave, or the duration of the Q wave is 0.04 second or more. A notched R wave may signify a bundle-branch block. A widened QRS complex (greater than 0.12 second) may signify a ventricular conduction delay. A missing QRS complex may indicate AV block or ventricular standstill.

LIFE STAGES ECG changes in an elderly adult may include increased PR interval, QRS duration, and QT interval, decreased amplitude of the QRS complex, and a shift of the QRS axis to the left.

ST SEGMENT

The ST segment represents the end of ventricular conduction or depolarization and the beginning of ventricular recovery or repolarization. The point that marks the end of the QRS complex and the beginning of the ST segment is known as the *J point.*

Pay special attention to the deflection of an ST segment. A normal ST segment has these characteristics (amplitude, duration, and configuration aren't observed):

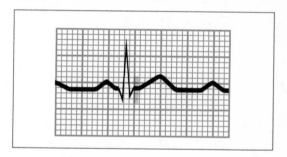

- location: extends from the S wave to the beginning of the T wave
- deflection: usually isoelectric (neither positive nor negative); may vary from −0.5 to +1 mm in some precordial leads.

depressed ST segment
ischemia or injury before infarcts dvps

Changes in the ST segment

Closely monitoring the ST segment on a patient's ECG can help you detect ischemia or injury before infarction develops.

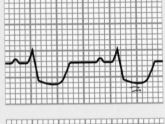

ST-SEGMENT DEPRESSION
An ST segment is considered depressed when it's 0.5 mm or more below the baseline. A depressed ST segment may indicate myocardial ischemia or digoxin toxicity.

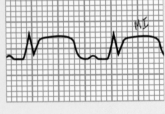

ST-SEGMENT ELEVATION
An ST segment is considered elevated when it's 1 mm or more above the baseline. An elevated ST segment may indicate myocardial injury.

ST segment changes
A change in the ST segment may indicate myocardial injury or ischemia. An ST segment may become either elevated or depressed. (See *Changes in the ST segment.*)

T WAVE
The peak of the T wave represents the relative refractory period of repolarization or ventricular recovery. When evaluating a T wave, look at the amplitude, configuration, and deflection.

Normal T waves have these characteristics (duration isn't measured):

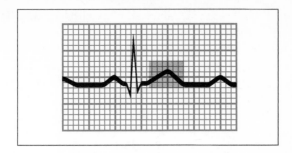

- location: follows the S wave
- amplitude: 0.5 mm in leads I, II, and III and up to 10 mm in the precordial leads
- configuration: typically rounded and smooth
- deflection: usually positive or upright in leads I, II, and V_3 to V_6; inverted in lead aV_R; variable in all other leads.

T-wave abnormalities

The T wave's peak represents the relative refractory period of ventricular repolarization, a period during which cells are especially vulnerable to extra stimuli. Bumps in a T wave may indicate that a P wave is hidden in it. If a P wave is hidden, atrial depolarization has occurred, the impulse having originated at a site above the ventricles.

Tall, peaked, or "tented" T waves may indicate myocardial injury or electrolyte imbalances such as hyperkalemia. Inverted T waves in leads I, II, or V_3 through V_6 may represent myocardial ischemia. Heavily notched or pointed T waves in an adult may mean pericarditis.

inverted T waves: Myocardial ischemia

QT INTERVAL

The QT interval measures the time needed for ventricular depolarization and repolarization. The length of the QT interval varies according to heart rate. The faster the heart rate, the shorter the QT interval. When checking the QT interval, look closely at the duration.

A normal QT interval has these characteristics (amplitude, configuration, and deflection aren't observed):

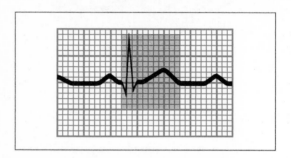

- location: extends from the beginning of the QRS complex to the end of the T wave
- duration: varies according to age, gender, and heart rate; usually lasts from 0.36 to 0.44 second; shouldn't be greater than half the distance between the two consecutive R waves (called the *R-R interval*) when the rhythm is regular.

QT wave variations

The QT interval measures the time needed for ventricular depolarization and repolarization. Prolonged QT intervals indicate that ventricular-repolarization time has slowed, meaning that the relative refractory or vulnerable period of the cardiac cycle is longer. (See *Correcting the QT interval.*)

This variation is also associated with certain drugs such as class I antiarrhythmics. Prolonged QT syndrome is a congenital conduction-system defect present in certain families. Short QT intervals may result from digoxin toxicity or electrolyte imbalances such as hypercalcemia.

Correcting the QT interval

The QT interval is affected by the patient's heart rate. As the heart rate increases, the QT interval decreases; as the heart rate decreases, the QT interval increases. For this reason, evaluating the QT interval based on a standard heart rate of 60 is recommended. This corrected QT interval is known as QTc. This formula is used to determine the QTc:

$$\frac{QT\ interval}{\sqrt{R\text{-}R\ interval\ in\ seconds}}$$

The normal QTc for women is less than 0.46 second and for men is less than 0.45 second. When the QTc is longer than 0.50 second in men or women, torsades de pointes is more likely to develop.

U WAVE

The U wave represents repolarization of the His-Purkinje system or ventricular conduction fibers. It isn't present on every rhythm strip. The configuration is the most important characteristic of the U wave.

When present, a normal U wave has these characteristics (amplitude and duration aren't measured):

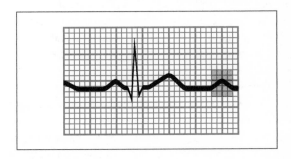

- location: follows the T wave
- configuration: typically upright and rounded
- deflection: upright.

U wave variations

The U wave may not appear on an ECG. A prominent U wave may be due to hypercalcemia, hypokalemia, or digoxin toxicity.

The 8-step method

Analyzing a rhythm strip is a skill developed through practice. You can use several methods, as long as you're consistent. Rhythm strip analysis requires a sequential and systematic approach such as using these eight steps.

STEP 1: DETERMINE RHYTHM

To determine the heart's atrial and ventricular rhythms, use either the paper-and-pencil method or the caliper method. (See *Methods of measuring rhythm.*)

Atrial rhythm determination

For atrial rhythm, measure the P-P intervals: the intervals between consecutive P waves. These intervals should occur regularly, with only small variations associated with respirations. Then compare the P-P intervals in several cycles. Consistently similar P-P intervals indicate regular atrial rhythm; dissimilar P-P intervals indicate irregular atrial rhythm.

Ventricular rhythm determination

To determine the ventricular rhythm, measure the intervals between two consecutive R waves in the QRS complexes. If an R wave isn't present, use either the Q wave or the S wave of consecutive QRS complexes. The R-R intervals should occur regularly. Then compare R-R intervals

Methods of measuring rhythm

You can use either of these methods to determine atrial or ventricular rhythm.

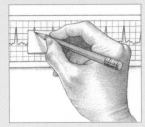

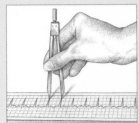

PAPER-AND-PENCIL METHOD
Place the ECG strip on a flat surface. Then position the straight edge of a piece of paper along the strip's baseline. Move the paper up slightly so the straight edge is near the peak of the R wave.

With a pencil, mark the paper at the R waves of two consecutive QRS complexes, as shown. This is the R-R interval. Next, move the paper across the strip lining up the two marks with succeeding R-R intervals. If the distance for each R-R interval is the same, the ventricular rhythm is regular. If the distance varies, the rhythm is irregular.

Use the same method to measure the distance between the P waves (the P-P interval) and determine whether the atrial rhythm is regular or irregular.

CALIPER METHOD
With the ECG on a flat surface, place one point of the calipers on the peak of the first R wave of two consecutive QRS complexes. Then adjust the caliper legs so the other point is on the peak of the next R wave, as shown. This distance is the R-R interval.

Now pivot the first point of the calipers toward the third R wave and note whether it falls on the peak of that wave. Check succeeding R-R intervals in the same way. If they're all the same, the ventricular rhythm is regular. If they vary, the rhythm is irregular.

Using the same method, measure the P-P intervals to determine whether the atrial rhythm is regular or irregular.

in several cycles. As with atrial rhythms, consistently similar intervals mean a regular rhythm; dissimilar intervals point to an irregular rhythm.

Rhythm analysis

After completing your measurements, ask yourself:

- Is the rhythm regular or irregular? Consider a rhythm with only slight variations, up to 0.04 second, to be regular.
- If the rhythm is irregular, is it slightly irregular or markedly so? Does the irregularity occur in a pattern (a regularly irregular pattern)?

STEP 2: CALCULATE RATE

You can use one of three methods to determine atrial and ventricular heart rates from an ECG waveform. Although these methods can provide accurate information, you shouldn't rely solely on them when assessing your patient. Keep in mind that the ECG waveform represents electrical, not mechanical, activity. Therefore, although an ECG can show you that ventricular depolarization has occurred, it doesn't mean that ventricular contraction has occurred. To do this, you must assess the patient's pulse. So remember, always check a pulse to correlate it with the heart rate on the ECG.

Times-ten method

The simplest, quickest, and most common way to calculate rate is the times-ten method, especially if the rhythm is irregular. ECG paper is marked in increments of 3 seconds, or 15 large boxes. To calculate the atrial rate:

- obtain a 6-second strip
- count the number of P waves on it
- multiply by 10. (Ten 6-second strips equal 1 minute.)

Calculate ventricular rate the same way, using the R waves.

1,500 method

If the heart rhythm is regular, use the 1,500 method, so named because 1,500 small squares equal 1 minute:

■ Count the number of small squares between identical points on two consecutive P waves.

■ Divide 1,500 by that number to get the atrial rate.

To obtain the ventricular rate, use the same method with two consecutive R waves.

Sequence method

The third method of estimating heart rate is the sequence method, which requires memorizing a sequence of numbers. (See *Calculating heart rate,* page 64.) For atrial rate:

■ find a P wave that peaks on a heavy black line and assign the following numbers to the next six heavy black lines: 300, 150, 100, 75, 60, and 50

■ find the next P wave peak

■ estimate the atrial rate, based on the number assigned to the nearest heavy black line.

Estimate the ventricular rate the same way, using the R wave.

STEP 3: EVALUATE P WAVE

When examining a rhythm strip for P waves, ask yourself:

■ Are P waves present?

■ Do the P waves have a normal configuration?

■ Do all the P waves have a similar size and shape?

■ Is there one P wave for every QRS complex?

STEP 4: DETERMINE PR-INTERVAL DURATION

To measure the PR interval, count the small squares between the start of the P wave and the start of the QRS complex; then multiply the number of squares by 0.04 second. After performing this calculation, ask yourself:

Calculating heart rate

This table can help make the sequencing method of determining heart rate more precise. After counting the number of boxes between the R waves, use this table to find the rate.

For example, if you count 20 small blocks or 4 large blocks, the rate would be 75 beats/minute. To calculate the atrial rate, use the same method with P waves instead of R waves.

RAPID ESTIMATION
This rapid-rate calculation is also called the *countdown method.* Using the number of large boxes between R waves or P waves as a guide, you can rapidly estimate ventricular or atrial rates by memorizing the sequence "300, 150, 100, 75, 60, 50."

NUMBER OF SMALL BLOCKS	HEART RATE
5 (1 large block)	300
6	250
7	214
8	187
9	166
10 (2 large blocks)	150
11	136
12	125
13	115
14	107
15 (3 large blocks)	100
16	94
17	88
18	83
19	79
20 (4 large blocks)	75
21	71
22	68
23	65
24	63
25 (5 large blocks)	60
26	58
27	56
28	54
29	52
30 (6 large blocks)	50
31	48
32	47
33	45
34	44
35 (7 large blocks)	43
36	41
37	40
38	39
39	38
40 (8 large blocks)	37

■ Does the duration of the PR interval fall within normal
limits, 0.12 to 0.20 second (or 3 to 5 small squares)?
■ Is the PR interval constant?

STEP 5: DETERMINE QRS-COMPLEX DURATION

When determining QRS-complex duration, make sure
you measure straight across from the end of the PR interval to the end of the S wave, not just to the peak. Remember, the QRS complex has no horizontal components. To
calculate duration, count the number of small squares between the beginning and end of the QRS complex and
multiply this number by 0.04 second. Then ask yourself:

■ Does the duration of the QRS complex fall within normal limits, 0.06 to 0.10 second?
■ Are all QRS complexes the same size and shape? (If
not, measure each one and describe them individually.)
■ Does a QRS complex appear after every P wave?

STEP 6: EVALUATE T WAVE

Examine the T waves on the ECG strip. Then ask yourself:
■ Are T waves present?
■ Do all of the T waves have a normal shape?
■ Could a P wave be hidden in a T wave?
■ Do all T waves have a normal amplitude?
■ Do the T waves have the same deflection as the QRS
complexes?

STEP 7: DETERMINE QT-INTERVAL DURATION

Count the number of small squares between the beginning of the QRS complex and the end of the T wave,
where the T wave returns to the baseline. Multiply this
number by 0.04 second. Ask yourself:

■ Does the duration of the QT interval fall within normal limits, 0.36 to 0.44 second?

STEP 8: EVALUATE OTHER COMPONENTS

Note the presence of ectopic or aberrantly conducted beats or other abnormalities. Also check the ST segment for abnormalities, and look for the presence of a U wave.

Now, interpret your findings by classifying the rhythm strip according to one or all of the following:

■ site of origin of the rhythm: for example, sinus node, atria, AV node, or ventricles

■ rate: normal (60 to 100 beats/ minute), bradycardia (less than 60 beats/minute), or tachycardia (greater than 100 beats/minute)

■ rhythm: normal or abnormal—for example, flutter, fibrillation, heart block, escape rhythm, or other arrhythmias.

Normal sinus rhythm

Before you can recognize an arrhythmia, you first need to be able to recognize normal sinus rhythm (NSR). NSR records an impulse that starts in the sinus node and progresses to the ventricles through a normal conduction pathway—from the sinus node to the atria and AV node, through the bundle of His, to the bundle branches, and on to the Purkinje fibers. There are no premature or aberrant contractions. NSR is the standard against which all other rhythms are compared. (See *Recognizing normal sinus rhythm.*)

The ECG characteristics of NSR include:

■ rhythm: regular atrial and ventricular rhythms

■ rate: atrial and ventricular rates 60 to 100 beats/minute, the SA node's normal firing rate

Recognizing normal sinus rhythm

Normal sinus rhythm (NSR), shown here, represents normal impulse conduction through the heart. This rhythm strip illustrates NSR.

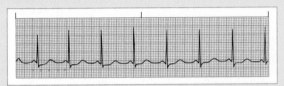

- *Rhythm:* atrial and ventricular rhythms regular
- *Rate:* atrial and ventricular rates normal, 80 beats/minute
- *P wave:* normal; precedes each QRS complex; all P waves similar in size and shape
- *PR interval:* normal, 0.12 second

- *QRS complex:* 0.06 second
- *T wave:* normal shape (upright and rounded)
- *QT interval:* normal, 0.40 second
- *Other:* no ectopic or aberrantly conducted impulses

- P waves: normally shaped (round and smooth) and upright in lead II; all P waves similar in size and shape; a P wave for every QRS complex
- PR interval: within normal limits (0.12 to 0.20 second)
- QRS complex: within normal limits (0.06 to 0.10 second)
- T wave: normally shaped; upright and rounded in lead II
- QT interval: within normal limits (0.36 to 0.44 second)
- Other: no ectopic or aberrant beats.

3

SINUS NODE ARRHYTHMIAS

When the heart functions normally, the sinoatrial (SA) node, also called the *sinus node,* acts as the primary pacemaker. The sinus node assumes this role because its automatic firing rate exceeds that of the heart's other pacemakers. In an adult at rest, the sinus node has an inherent firing rate of 60 to 100 times per minute.

In about 55% of people, the SA node's blood supply comes from the right coronary artery, and in about 45% of people, it comes from the left circumflex artery. The autonomic nervous system (ANS) richly innervates the sinus node through the vagus nerve, a parasympathetic nerve, and several sympathetic nerves. Stimulation of the vagus nerve decreases the node's firing rate, and stimulation of the sympathetic system increases it.

Changes in the automaticity of the sinus node or in its blood supply, and ANS influences may all lead to sinus node arrhythmias. This chapter will help you to identify sinus node arrhythmias on an electrocardiogram (ECG). It will also help you to determine the causes, significance, signs and symptoms, treatment, and interventions associated with each arrhythmia presented.

The 8-step method to analyze the ECG strip will be used for each of the arrhythmias described.

Sinus arrhythmia

In sinus arrhythmia, the rate stays within normal limits but the rhythm is irregular and corresponds to the respiratory cycle, accelerating with inspiration and slowing with expiration. Sinus arrhythmia can occur normally in athletes, children, and older adults, but it rarely occurs in infants. Conditions unrelated to respiration that may also produce sinus arrhythmia include:

- heart disease
- old age
- inferior wall myocardial infarction (MI)
- the use of certain drugs, such as digoxin and morphine
- increased intracranial pressure (ICP).

CAUSES

Sinus arrhythmia, the heart's normal response to respirations, results from an inhibition of reflex vagal activity, or tone. During inspiration, an increase in the flow of blood back to the heart reduces vagal tone, which increases the heart rate. ECG complexes fall closer together, which shortens the P-P interval. During expiration, venous return decreases, which in turn increases vagal tone, slows the heart rate, and lengthens the P-P interval. (See *Recognizing sinus arrhythmia,* page 70.)

CLINICAL SIGNIFICANCE

Sinus arrhythmia usually isn't significant and produces no symptoms. A marked variation in P-P intervals in an elderly adult, however, may indicate sick sinus syndrome (SSS)—a related, potentially more serious phenomenon.

ECG CHARACTERISTICS

- *Rhythm:* Atrial rhythm is irregular, corresponding to the respiratory cycle. The P-P interval is shorter during in-

Recognizing sinus arrhythmia

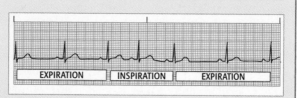

This rhythm strip illustrates sinus arrhythmia.

- *Rhythm:* cyclic, irregular; varies with respiratory cycle
- *Rate:* 70 beats/minute
- *P wave:* normal
- *PR interval:* 0.16 second
- *QRS complex:* 0.06 second
- *T wave:* normal
- *QT interval:* 0.36 second
- *Other:* phasic slowing and quickening

spiration, longer during expiration. The difference between the longest and shortest P-P interval exceeds 0.12 second. Ventricular rhythm is also irregular, corresponding to the respiratory cycle. The R-R interval is shorter during inspiration, longer during expiration. The difference between the longest and shortest R-R interval exceeds 0.12 second.

- *Rate:* Atrial and ventricular rates are within normal limits (60 to 100 beats/minute) and vary with respiration. Typically, the heart rate increases during inspiration and decreases during expiration.
- *P wave:* Normal size and configuration; P wave precedes each QRS complex.
- *PR interval:* May vary slightly within normal limits.
- *QRS complex:* Normal duration and configuration.
- *T wave:* Normal size and configuration.
- *QT interval:* May vary slightly but is usually within normal limits.
- *Other:* None.

SIGNS AND SYMPTOMS

The patient may exhibit peripheral pulse rate increases during inspiration and decreases during expiration. Sinus arrhythmia is easier to detect when the heart rate is slow; it may disappear when the heart rate increases, as with exercise.

If the arrhythmia is caused by an underlying condition, you may note signs and symptoms of that condition. Marked sinus arrhythmia may cause dizziness or syncope in some cases.

TREATMENT

Unless the patient is symptomatic, treatment usually isn't necessary. If sinus arrhythmia is unrelated to respirations, the underlying cause may require treatment.

NURSING INTERVENTIONS

When caring for a patient with sinus arrhythmia:

- Monitor the heart rhythm during respiration to determine whether the arrhythmia coincides with the respiratory cycle.
- Check the rhythm carefully to avoid an inaccurate interpretation of the waveform.
- If induced by drugs, such as morphine sulfate and other sedatives, notify the practitioner, who will decide whether to continue the drugs.

RED FLAG If sinus arrhythmia develops suddenly in a patient taking digoxin, assess for signs of digoxin toxicity, such as nausea, ringing in the ears, and changes in mental status. If these occur, notify the practitioner immediately.

Recognizing sinus bradycardia

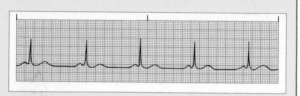

This rhythm strip illustrates sinus bradycardia.

- Rhythm: regular
- *Rate:* 50 beats/minute
- *P wave:* normal; precedes each QRS complex
- *PR interval:* 0.16 second
- *QRS complex:* 0.08 second
- *T wave:* normal
- *QT interval:* 0.50 second
- *Other:* none

Sinus bradycardia

Sinus bradycardia is characterized by a sinus rate below 60 beats/minute and a regular rhythm. All impulses originate in the SA node. This arrhythmia's significance depends on the symptoms and the underlying cause. (See *Recognizing sinus bradycardia.*)

CAUSES

Sinus bradycardia usually occurs as the normal response to a reduced demand for blood flow. In this case, vagal stimulation increases and sympathetic stimulation decreases. As a result, automaticity (the tendency of cells to initiate their own impulses) in the SA node diminishes. It may occur normally during sleep or in a person with a well-conditioned heart, such as an athlete.

Sinus bradycardia may be caused by:

- noncardiac disorders, such as hyperkalemia, increased ICP, hypothyroidism, hypothermia, and glaucoma
- conditions producing excess vagal stimulation or decreased sympathetic stimulation, such as sleep, deep relaxation, the Valsalva maneuver, carotid sinus massage, and vomiting
- cardiac diseases, such as SA node disease, cardiomyopathy, myocarditis, myocardial ischemia, and heart block; can also occur immediately following an inferior wall MI that involves the right coronary artery, which supplies blood to the SA node.
- certain drugs, especially beta blockers, digoxin, calcium channel blockers, lithium, and antiarrhythmics, such as sotalol, amiodarone, propafenone, and quinidine.

CLINICAL SIGNIFICANCE

The significance of sinus bradycardia depends on how low the rate is and whether the patient is symptomatic. For example, most adults can tolerate a sinus bradycardia of 45 to 59 beats/minute but are less tolerant of a rate below 45 beats/minute.

Typically, sinus bradycardia is asymptomatic and insignificant. Many athletes develop sinus bradycardia because their well-conditioned hearts can maintain a normal stroke volume with less-than-normal effort. Sinus bradycardia also occurs normally during sleep as a result of circadian variations in heart rate.

RED FLAG When sinus bradycardia is symptomatic, however, prompt attention is critical. The heart of a patient with underlying cardiac disease may be unable to compensate for a drop in rate by increasing its stroke volume. The resulting drop in cardiac output produces signs and symptoms, such as hypotension and dizziness. Bradycardia may also predispose some patients to more

‿ bad

*serious arrhythmias, such as ventricular tachycardia and
ventricular fibrillation.* V-Fib

ECG CHARACTERISTICS

■ *Rhythm:* Atrial and ventricular rhythms are regular.
■ *Rate:* Atrial and ventricular rates are less than
  60 beats/minute.
■ *P wave:* Normal size and configuration; P wave pre-
  cedes each QRS complex.
■ *PR interval:* Within normal limits and constant.
■ *QRS complex:* Normal duration and configuration.
■ *T wave:* Normal size and configuration.
■ *QT interval:* Within normal limits but may be pro-
  longed.
■ *Other:* None.

SIGNS AND SYMPTOMS

The patient will have a pulse rate of less than 60 beats/
minute, with a regular rhythm. As long as he's able to
compensate for the decreased cardiac output, he'll likely
stay asymptomatic. If compensatory mechanisms fail,
however, signs and symptoms of declining cardiac output
usually appear, including:
■ altered mental status
■ blurred vision
■ chest pain
■ cool, clammy skin
■ crackles, dyspnea, and an S_3, or third heart sound, indicating heart failure
■ dizziness
■ hypotension
■ syncope.

   Palpitations and pulse irregularities may occur if the
patient experiences ectopy such as premature atrial, junctional, or ventricular contractions. This is because the SA

node's increased relative refractory period permits ectopic firing. Bradycardia-induced syncope (Stokes-Adams attack) may also occur.

TREATMENT
If the patient is asymptomatic and his vital signs are stable, treatment generally isn't necessary. If the patient is symptomatic, treatment aims to identify and correct the underlying cause. (See ACLS bradycardia algorithm, page 260.)

NURSING INTERVENTIONS
■ Observe the patient, and monitor the progression and duration of the bradycardia.
■ Evaluate the patient's tolerance of the rhythm at rest and with activity.
■ Review the patient's drugs, and check with the practitioner about stopping drugs that may be depressing the SA node, such as digoxin, beta blockers, or calcium channel blockers.
■ Prepare the patient for treatments, such as drug administration (atropine, dopamine, epinephrine) or temporary or permanent pacemaker insertion.

Sinus tachycardia

Sinus tachycardia is accelerated firing of the SA node beyond its normal discharge rate. Sinus tachycardia in an adult is characterized by a sinus rate of more than 100 beats/minute. The rate rarely exceeds 180 beats/minute except during strenuous exercise; the maximum rate achievable with exercise decreases with age. (See *Recognizing sinus tachycardia,* page 76.)

Recognizing sinus tachycardia

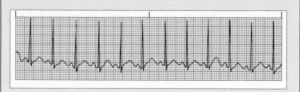

This rhythm strip illustrates sinus tachycardia.

- *Rhythm:* regular
- *Rate:* 120 beats/minute
- *P wave:* normal; precedes each QRS complex
- *PR interval:* 0.14 second
- *QRS complex:* 0.06 second
- *T wave:* normal
- *QT interval:* 0.34 second
- *Other:* none

CAUSES

Sinus tachycardia may be a normal response to exercise, pain, stress, fever, or strong emotions, such as fear and anxiety. Other causes of sinus tachycardia include:

- cardiac conditions, such as heart failure, cardiogenic shock, and pericarditis
- drugs, such as atropine, isoproterenol, aminophylline, dopamine, dobutamine, epinephrine, alcohol, caffeine, nicotine, and amphetamines
- other conditions, such as shock, anemia, respiratory distress, pulmonary embolism, sepsis, and hyperthyroidism, where the increased heart rate serves as a compensatory mechanism.

CLINICAL SIGNIFICANCE

The significance of sinus tachycardia depends on the underlying cause. The arrhythmia may be the body's response to exercise or high emotional states and of no clinical significance. It may also occur with anxiety, fear, hypovolemia, hemorrhage, or pain. When the stimulus for the tachycardia is removed, the arrhythmia generally resolves spontaneously.

Although sinus tachycardia commonly occurs without serious signs and symptoms, persistent sinus tachycardia can also be serious, especially if it occurs in the setting of an acute MI. Tachycardia can lower cardiac output by reducing ventricular filling time and stroke volume. Normally, ventricular volume reaches 120 to 130 ml during diastole. In tachycardia, decreased ventricular volume leads to decreased cardiac output with subsequent hypotension and decreased peripheral perfusion.

Tachycardia worsens myocardial ischemia by increasing the heart's demand for oxygen and reducing the duration of diastole, the period of greatest coronary blood flow.

An increase in heart rate can also be detrimental for patients with obstructive types of heart conditions, such as aortic stenosis and hypertrophic cardiomyopathy. Persistent tachycardia may also signal impending heart failure or cardiogenic shock. Sinus tachycardia can also cause angina in patients with coronary artery disease.

ECG CHARACTERISTICS

- *Rhythm:* Atrial and ventricular rhythms are regular.
- *Rate:* Atrial and ventricular rates are greater than 100 beats/minute, usually between 100 and 160 beats/minute.
- *P wave:* Normal size and configuration, but it may increase in amplitude. A P wave precedes each QRS complex, but as the heart rate increases, the P wave may be superimposed on the preceding T wave and difficult to identify.
- *PR interval:* Within normal limits and constant.
- *QRS complex:* Normal duration and configuration.

- *T wave:* Normal size and configuration.
- *QT interval:* Within normal limits but commonly shortened.
- *Other:* None.

SIGNS AND SYMPTOMS
The patient will have a peripheral pulse rate above 100 beats/minute but a regular rhythm. Typically, he'll be asymptomatic. However, if his cardiac output falls and compensatory mechanisms fail, he may experience:
- hypotension
- syncope
- blurred vision
- chest pain and palpitations
- nervousness or anxiety.

If heart failure develops, he may exhibit crackles, an extra heart sound (S_3), and jugular vein distention.

TREATMENT
When treating the asymptomatic patient, focus is on determining the cause of the tachycardia. The focus of treatment in the symptomatic patient with sinus tachycardia is to maintain adequate cardiac output and tissue perfusion and to identify and correct the underlying cause. For example, if tachycardia is caused by hemorrhage, treatment includes stopping the bleeding and replacing blood and fluid losses.

If tachycardia leads to cardiac ischemia, treatment may include drugs to slow the heart rate. The most commonly used drugs include beta blockers, such as metoprolol and atenolol, and calcium channel blockers such as verapamil.

NURSING INTERVENTIONS

■ Check the patient's medication history. Over-the-counter sympathomimetics, which mimic the effects of the sympathetic nervous system, may contribute to the sinus tachycardia. Sympathomimetics may be contained in nose drops and cold formulas.

■ Question the patient about his use of caffeine, nicotine, and alcohol, each of which can trigger tachycardia. Advise him to avoid these substances.

■ Ask the patient about his use of illicit drugs, such as cocaine and amphetamines, which can also cause tachycardia.

■ Assess the patient for signs and symptoms of angina and heart failure.

■ Monitor intake and output, along with daily weight.

■ Check the patient's level of consciousness to assess cerebral perfusion.

■ Provide a calm environment. Help to reduce the patient's fear and anxiety, which can aggravate his arrhythmia.

■ Teach about procedures and treatments. Include relaxation techniques in the information you provide.

■ Tachycardia is frequently the initial sign of pulmonary embolism. Stay alert to this possibility, especially if your patient has predisposing risk factors for thrombotic emboli.

RED FLAG Be aware that a sudden onset of sinus tachycardia after an MI may signal extension of the infarction. Notify the practitioner promptly.

Sinus arrest and sinoatrial exit block

Although sinus arrest and SA or sinus exit block are two separate arrhythmias with different etiologies, they're dis-

Recognizing sinus arrest

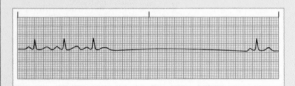

This rhythm strip illustrates sinus arrest.

- *Rhythm:* regular, except for the missing PQRST complexes
- *Rate:* underlying rhythm, 75 beats/minute
- *P wave:* normal; missing during pause
- *PR interval:* 0.20 second
- *QRS complex:* 0.08 second; missing during pause
- *T wave:* normal; missing during pause
- *QT interval:* 0.40 second; missing during pause
- *Other:* none

cussed together because distinguishing the two is typically difficult. Also, there's no difference in their clinical significance and treatment.

In sinus arrest, the normal sinus rhythm is interrupted by an occasional, prolonged failure of the SA node to initiate an impulse. Therefore, sinus arrest is caused by episodes of failure in the automaticity or impulse formation of the SA node. The atria aren't stimulated, and an entire PQRST complex is missing from the ECG strip. Except for this missing complex, or pause, the ECG usually remains normal. When one or two impulses aren't formed, it's called a *sinus pause;* when three or more impulses aren't formed, it's called a *sinus arrest.* (See *Recognizing sinus arrest.*)

In SA exit block, the SA node discharges at regular intervals but some impulses are delayed or blocked from reaching the atria, resulting in long sinus pauses. Blocks

Recognizing sinoatrial exit block

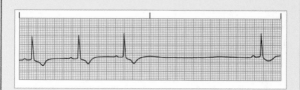

This rhythm strip illustrates sinoatrial (SA) exit block.

- *Rhythm:* regular, except for pauses
- *Rate:* underlying rhythm, 60 beats/minute before SA block; length or frequency of the pause may result in bradycardia
- *P wave:* periodically absent
- *PR interval:* 0.16 second
- *QRS complex:* 0.08 second; missing during pause
- *T wave:* normal; missing during pause
- *QT interval:* 0.40 second; missing during pause
- *Other:* entire PQRST complex missing; pause ends with sinus rhythm or atrial escape rhythm

result from failure to conduct impulses, while sinus arrest results from failure to form impulses in the SA node. Both arrhythmias cause atrial activity to stop. In sinus arrest, the pause commonly ends with a junctional escape beat. In SA exit block, the pause occurs for an indefinite period and ends with a sinus rhythm. (See *Recognizing sinoatrial exit block.*)

CAUSES

Causes of sinus arrest and SA exit block include:
- acute infection
- cardiac disorders, such as coronary artery disease, acute myocarditis, cardiomyopathy, hypertensive heart disease, and acute inferior wall MI

- digoxin, quinidine, procainamide, and salicylate toxicity
- excessive doses of beta blockers, such as metoprolol and propranolol
- increased vagal tone, such as with the Valsalva maneuver, carotid sinus massage, and vomiting
- sick sinus syndrome (SSS)
- sinus node disease, such as fibrosis and idiopathic degeneration.

CLINICAL SIGNIFICANCE

The significance of these two arrhythmias depends on the patient's symptoms. If the pauses are short and infrequent, the patient will most likely be asymptomatic and not require treatment. He may have a normal sinus rhythm for days or weeks between episodes of sinus arrest or SA exit block, and he may be totally unaware of the arrhythmia. Pauses of 2 to 3 seconds normally occur in healthy adults during sleep, and occasionally in patients with increased vagal tone or hypersensitive carotid sinus disease.

If either arrhythmia is frequent or prolonged, however, the patient will most likely experience symptoms related to low cardiac output. The arrhythmias can produce syncope or near-syncopal episodes usually within 7 seconds of asystole.

RED FLAG *During a prolonged pause, the patient may fall and injure himself. Other situations are potentially just as serious. For example, a symptomatic arrhythmia that occurs while the patient is driving a car could result in a fatal accident. Extremely slow rates can also give rise to other arrhythmias.*

ECG CHARACTERISTICS

Both sinus arrest and SA exit block share these ECG characteristics:

- *Rhythm:* Atrial and ventricular rhythms are usually regular except for when sinus arrest or SA exit block occurs.
- *Rate:* The underlying atrial and ventricular rates are usually within normal limits (60 to 100 beats/minute) before the arrest or SA exit block occurs. The length or frequency of the pause may result in bradycardia.
- *P wave:* Periodically absent, with entire PQRST complex missing. However, when present, the P wave is normal in size and configuration and precedes each QRS complex.
- *PR interval:* Within normal limits and constant when a P wave is present.
- *QRS complex:* Normal duration and configuration but absent during a pause.
- *T wave:* Normal size and configuration but absent during a pause.
- *QT interval:* Usually within normal limits but absent during a pause.

Differentiation criteria

To differentiate between these two rhythms, compare the length of the pause with the underlying P-P or R-R interval. If the underlying rhythm is regular, determine whether the underlying rhythm resumes on time after the pause. With SA exit block, because the regularity of the SA node discharge is blocked, not interrupted, the underlying rhythm will resume on time following the pause. In addition, the length of the pause will be a multiple of the underlying P-P or R-R interval.

In sinus arrest, the timing of the SA node discharge is interrupted by the failure of the SA node to initiate an impulse. The result is that the underlying rhythm doesn't resume on time after the pause and the length of the pause is not a multiple of the previous R-R intervals.

SIGNS AND SYMPTOMS

You won't be able to detect a pulse or heart sounds when sinus arrest or SA exit block occurs. Short pauses usually produce no symptoms, and the patient is asymptomatic. Recurrent or prolonged pauses may cause signs of decreased cardiac output, such as:

■ low blood pressure
■ altered mental status
■ cool, clammy skin
■ syncopal episodes
■ dizziness or blurred vision.

TREATMENT

An asymptomatic patient needs no treatment. Symptomatic patients are treated following the guidelines for patients with symptomatic bradycardia. (See Bradycardia algorithm, page 260.) Treatment will also focus on the cause of the sinus arrest or SA exit block. This may involve stopping drugs that contribute to SA node discharge or conduction, such as digoxin, beta blockers, and calcium channel blockers.

NURSING INTERVENTIONS

■ Monitor the heart rhythm.
■ Protect the patient from injury, such as a fall, which may result from a syncopal or near-syncopal pause.
■ If pauses are recurrent, assess the patient for evidence of decreased cardiac output, such as altered mental status, low blood pressure, and cool, clammy skin.
■ Document the patient's vital signs and how he feels during pauses as well as the activities he was involved in at the time.
■ Assess for a progression of the arrhythmia. Notify the practitioner immediately if the patient becomes unstable.

■ Be alert for signs of digoxin, quinidine, or procainamide toxicity. Obtain digoxin and electrolyte levels.

Sick sinus syndrome

Also known as *SA syndrome, sinus nodal dysfunction,* and *Stokes-Adams syndrome,* SSS refers to a wide spectrum of SA node arrhythmias. It's caused by disturbances in the way impulses are generated or in the ability to conduct impulses to the atria. These disturbances may be either intrinsic or mediated by the ANS.

SSS usually shows up as bradycardia, with episodes of sinus arrest and SA exit block interspersed with sudden, brief periods of rapid atrial fibrillation. Patients are also prone to paroxysms of other atrial tachyarrhythmias, such as atrial flutter and ectopic atrial tachycardia, a condition sometimes referred to as *bradycardia-tachycardia* (or *brady-tachy) syndrome.*

Most patients with SSS are older than age 60, but anyone can develop the arrhythmia. It's rare in children except after open-heart surgery that results in SA node damage. The arrhythmia affects men and women equally; onset is progressive, insidious, and chronic. (See *Recognizing sick sinus syndrome,* page 86.)

CAUSES

SSS results either from a dysfunction of the sinus node's automaticity or from abnormal conduction or blockages of impulses coming out of the nodal region. These conditions, in turn, stem from a degeneration of the area's ANS and partial destruction of the sinus node, as may occur with an interrupted blood supply after an inferior wall MI.

Recognizing sick sinus syndrome

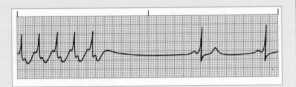

This rhythm strip illustrates sick sinus syndrome.

- *Rhythm:* irregular
- *Rate:* atrial and ventricular rates fast (150 beats/minute) or slow (43 beats/minute) or alternate between fast and slow; interrupted by a long sinus pause
- *P wave:* varies with prevailing rhythm
- *PR interval:* varies with rhythm
- *QRS complex:* 0.10 second; may vary with rhythm
- *T wave:* configuration varies
- *QT interval:* varies with rhythm changes
- *Other:* sinus pause due to nonfiring sinus node

Also, certain conditions can affect the atrial wall surrounding the SA node and cause exit blocks. Conditions that cause inflammation or degeneration of atrial tissue can also lead to SSS. In many patients, however, the exact cause is never identified.

Causes of SSS include:

- conditions leading to fibrosis of the SA node, such as increased age, atherosclerotic heart disease, hypertension, ischemia, MI, and cardiomyopathy
- trauma to the SA node caused by open-heart surgery (especially valvular surgery), pericarditis, or rheumatic heart disease
- autonomic disturbances affecting autonomic innervation, such as increased vagal tone or degeneration of the autonomic system

■ cardioactive drugs, such as digoxin, beta blockers, and calcium channel blockers.

CLINICAL SIGNIFICANCE

The significance of SSS depends on the patient's age, the presence of other diseases, and the type and duration of the specific arrhythmias that occur. If atrial fibrillation is involved, the prognosis is worse, most likely because of the risk of thromboembolic complications.

If prolonged pauses are involved with SSS, syncope may occur. The length of a pause needed to cause syncope varies with the patient's age, posture at the time, and cerebrovascular status. A pause that lasts 2 to 3 seconds or more is considered significant.

A significant part of the diagnosis is whether the patient experiences symptoms while the disturbance occurs. Because the syndrome is progressive and chronic, a symptomatic patient will need lifelong treatment. In addition, thromboembolism may develop as a complication of SSS, possibly resulting in stroke or peripheral embolization.

ECG CHARACTERISTICS

SSS encompasses several potential rhythm disturbances that may be intermittent or chronic. It includes one or a combination of these rhythm disturbances:

■ sinus bradycardia
■ SA block
■ sinus arrest
■ sinus bradycardia alternating with sinus tachycardia
■ episodes of atrial tachyarrhythmias, such as atrial fibrillation and atrial flutter
■ failure of the sinus node to increase heart rate with exercise.

SSS displays these ECG characteristics:

- *Rhythm:* Atrial and ventricular rhythms irregular because of sinus pauses and abrupt rate changes.
- *Rate:* Atrial and ventricular rates fast or slow, or alternate between fast and slow; and interrupted by a long sinus pause.
- *P wave:* Varies with the prevailing rhythm; may be normal size and configuration or may be absent; when present, a P wave usually precedes each QRS complex.
- *PR interval:* Usually within normal limits; varies with change in rhythm.
- *QRS complex:* Duration usually within normal limits; may vary with changes in rhythm; usually normal configuration.
- *T wave:* Usually normal size and configuration.
- *QT interval:* Usually within normal limits; varies with rhythm changes.
- *Other:* Usually more than one arrhythmia on a 6-second strip.

SIGNS AND SYMPTOMS

The patient's pulse rate may be fast, slow, or normal, and the rhythm may be regular or irregular. You can usually detect an irregularity on the monitor or when palpating the pulse, which may feel inappropriately slow then rapid.

If you monitor the patient's heart rate during exercise or exertion, you may observe an inappropriate response to exercise, such as:

- failure of the heart rate to increase
- brady-tachy syndrome
- atrial flutter
- atrial fibrillation
- SA block
- sinus arrest on the monitor.

Other assessment findings depend on the patient's condition. For example, he may have crackles in the lungs, S_3, or a dilated and displaced left ventricular apical impulse if he has underlying cardiomyopathy.

The patient may also show signs and symptoms of decreased cardiac output, such as:

■ fatigue

■ hypotension

■ blurred vision

■ syncope, a common experience with this arrhythmia.

LIFE STAGES Because the older adult with SSS may have mental status changes, make sure you perform a thorough assessment to rule out such disorders as stroke, delirium, or dementia.

TREATMENT

As with other sinus node arrhythmias, no treatment is generally necessary if the patient is asymptomatic. If the patient is symptomatic, however, treatment aims to relieve signs and symptoms and correct the underlying cause of the arrhythmia.

Atropine or epinephrine may be given initially for symptomatic bradycardia. (See Bradycardia algorithm, page 260.) A temporary pacemaker may be required until the underlying disorder resolves. Tachyarrhythmias may be treated with antiarrhythmics, such as metoprolol and digoxin. Unfortunately, drugs used to suppress tachyarrhythmias may worsen underlying SA node disease and bradyarrhythmias.

The patient may need anticoagulants if he develops sudden bursts, or paroxysms, of atrial fibrillation. The anticoagulants help prevent thromboembolism and stroke, complications of the condition.

NURSING INTERVENTIONS

■ Monitor and document all arrhythmias as well as signs or symptoms experienced.

■ Note changes in heart rate and rhythm related to changes in the patient's level of activity.

■ Look for signs and symptoms of thromboembolism, especially if the patient has atrial fibrillation. Blood clots or thrombi forming in the heart can dislodge and travel through the bloodstream, resulting in decreased blood supply to the lungs, heart, brain, kidneys, intestines, or other organs.

■ Assess the patient for neurologic changes, such as confusion, vision disturbances, weakness, chest pain, dyspnea, tachypnea, tachycardia, and acute onset of pain. Early recognition allows for prompt treatment.

■ Watch the patient carefully after starting beta blockers and calcium channel blockers, or other antiarrhythmics.

■ Prepare the patient for possible treatment interventions, such as anticoagulant therapy and pacemaker insertion.

4

ATRIAL ARRHYTHMIAS

Atrial arrhythmias, the most common cardiac rhythm disturbances, result from impulses originating in the atrial tissue outside of the sinoatrial (SA) node. These arrhythmias can affect ventricular filling time and diminish atrial kick. The term *atrial kick* refers to the complete filling of the ventricles during atrial systole. Atrial kick accounts for 15% to 25% of cardiac output in healthy adults and up to 50% of cardiac output in those with decreased ventricular compliance. The loss of atrial kick may significantly decrease cardiac output and produce signs and symptoms of decreased perfusion in some patients.

Atrial arrhythmias probably result from three mechanisms:

- *Altered automaticity.* The term *automaticity* refers to the ability of cardiac cells to initiate electrical impulses spontaneously. An increase in the automaticity of the atrial fibers can trigger abnormal impulses. Causes of increased automaticity include extracellular factors, such as hypoxia, hypocalcemia, and digoxin toxicity, as well as conditions in which the function of the heart's normal pacemaker, the SA node, is diminished. For example, increased vagal tone or hypokalemia can increase the refractory period of the SA node and allow atrial fibers to initiate impulses.
- *Reentry.* In reentry, an impulse is delayed along a slow conduction pathway. Despite the delay, the impulse

remains active enough to produce another impulse during myocardial repolarization, resulting in an abnormal continuous circuit. Reentry may occur with coronary artery disease (CAD), cardiomyopathy, or myocardial infarction (MI) and is the most common mechanism in atrial arrhythmias.

■ *Afterdepolarization.* Afterdepolarization can occur as a result of cell injury, digoxin toxicity, and other conditions. An injured cell sometimes only partially repolarizes. Partial repolarization can lead to repetitive ectopic firing called *triggered activity.* The depolarization produced by triggered activity, known as *afterdepolarization,* can lead to atrial or ventricular tachycardia.

This chapter will help you identify atrial arrhythmias, including premature atrial contractions (PACs), atrial tachycardia, atrial flutter, atrial fibrillation, Ashman's phenomenon, and wandering pacemaker. The chapter reviews causes, clinical significance, electrocardiogram (ECG) characteristics, and signs and symptoms of each arrhythmia as well as interventions directed at treating the patient experiencing these arrhythmias.

Premature atrial contractions

PACs originate in the atria, outside the SA node. They arise from either a single ectopic focus or from multiple atrial foci that supersede the SA node as pacemaker for one or more beats. PACs are generally caused by enhanced automaticity in the atrial tissue. (See *Recognizing PACs.*)

PACs may be conducted or nonconducted (blocked) through the atrioventricular (AV) node and the rest of the heart, depending on the status of the AV and intraventricular conduction system. If the atrial ectopic pacemaker discharges too early after the preceding QRS complex, the

Recognizing PACs

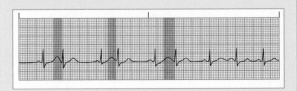

This rhythm strip illustrates sinus rhythm with premature atrial contractions (PACs).

- Rhythm: irregular
- *Rate:* 90 beats/minute
- *P wave:* premature and abnormally shaped with PACs (see shaded areas)
- *PR interval:* 0.12 to 0.18 second for the underlying

rhythm; unmeasurable for the PAC
- *QRS complex:* 0.08 second
- *T wave:* abnormal with embedded P waves of PACs
- *QT interval:* 0.32 second
- *Other:* compensatory pause

AV junction or bundle branches may still be refractory from conducting the previous electrical impulse. If they're still refractory, they may not be sufficiently repolarized to conduct the premature electrical impulse into the ventricles normally.

When a PAC is conducted, ventricular conduction is usually normal. Nonconducted, or blocked, PACs aren't followed by a QRS complex.

CAUSES

Alcohol, cigarettes, anxiety, fatigue, caffeine, fever, and infectious diseases can trigger PACs, which commonly occur in a normal heart. Patients who eliminate or control those factors can usually correct the arrhythmia.

PACs may be associated with:
■ hyperthyroidism

- coronary or valvular heart disease
- acute respiratory failure
- hypoxia
- chronic obstructive pulmonary disease (COPD)
- digoxin toxicity
- certain electrolyte imbalances.

PACs may be caused by drugs that prolong the absolute refractory period of the SA node, including quinidine and procainamide. Endogenous catecholamine release during episodes of pain or anxiety may also cause PACs.

CLINICAL SIGNIFICANCE

PACs are rarely dangerous in patients free from heart disease. They often cause no symptoms and can go unrecognized for years. Patients may perceive PACs as normal palpitations or skipped beats.

However, in patients with heart disease, PACs may lead to more serious arrhythmias, such as atrial fibrillation or atrial flutter.

RED FLAG In a patient with acute MI, PACs can serve as an early sign of heart failure or electrolyte imbalance.

ECG CHARACTERISTICS

- *Rhythm:* Atrial and ventricular rhythms are irregular as a result of PACs, but the underlying rhythm may be regular.
- *Rate:* Atrial and ventricular rates vary with the underlying rhythm.
- *P wave:* The hallmark characteristic of a PAC is a premature P wave with an abnormal configuration, when compared with a sinus P wave. Varying configurations of the P wave indicate more than one ectopic site. PACs may be hidden in the preceding T wave.

■ *PR interval:* Usually within normal limits but may be either shortened or slightly prolonged for the ectopic beat, depending on the origin of the ectopic focus.

■ *QRS complex:* Duration and configuration are usually normal when the PAC is conducted. If no QRS complex follows the PAC, the beat is called a *nonconducted PAC*.

■ *T wave:* Usually normal; however, if the P wave is hidden in the T wave, the T wave may appear distorted.

■ *QT interval:* Usually within normal limits.

■ *Other:* PACs may occur as a single beat, in a bigeminal (every other beat is premature), trigeminal (every third beat), or quadrigeminal (every fourth beat) pattern, or in couplets (pairs). Three or more PACs in a row are called *atrial tachycardia*.

PACs are commonly followed by a pause as the SA node resets. The PAC depolarizes the SA node early, causing it to reset itself and disrupting the normal cycle. The next sinus beat occurs sooner than it normally would, causing a P-P interval between normal beats interrupted by a PAC to be shorter than three consecutive sinus beats, an occurrence referred to as *noncompensatory*.

SIGNS AND SYMPTOMS

The patient may have an irregular peripheral or apical pulse rhythm when the PACs occur. Otherwise, the pulse rhythm and rate will reflect the underlying rhythm. Patients may complain of palpitations, skipped beats, or a fluttering sensation. In a patient with heart disease, signs and symptoms of decreased cardiac output, such as hypotension and syncope, may occur.

TREATMENT

Most asymptomatic patients don't need treatment. If the patient is symptomatic, however, treatment may focus on eliminating the cause, such as caffeine and alcohol. People with frequent PACs may be treated with drugs that prolong the refractory period of the atria. Those drugs include digoxin and beta and calcium channel blockers.

NURSING INTERVENTIONS

■ Assess the patient to help determine factors that trigger ectopic beats.

■ If the patient has ischemic or valvular heart disease, monitor for signs and symptoms of heart failure, electrolyte imbalance, and more severe atrial arrhythmias.

■ Teach the patient to correct or avoid underlying causes. For example, the patient might need to avoid caffeine or learn stress reduction techniques to lessen anxiety.

Atrial tachycardia

Atrial tachycardia is a supraventricular tachycardia, which means that the impulses driving the rapid rhythm originate above the ventricles. Atrial tachycardia has an atrial rate from 150 to 250 beats/minute. The rapid rate shortens diastole, resulting in a loss of atrial kick, reduced cardiac output, reduced coronary perfusion, and the potential for myocardial ischemia. (See *Recognizing atrial tachycardia.*)

Three forms of atrial tachycardia are discussed here:

■ atrial tachycardia with block

■ multifocal atrial tachycardia (MAT), also known as *chaotic atrial tachycardia*

■ paroxysmal atrial tachycardia (PAT).

In atrial tachycardia with block, not all atrial impulses are conducted through to the ventricles. In MAT, the tachycardia originates from multiple atrial foci. PAT is generally a transient event in which the tachycardia appears and disappears suddenly.

Recognizing atrial tachycardia

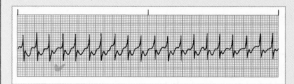

This rhythm strip illustrates atrial tachycardia.

- *Rhythm:* regular
- *Rate:* 200 beats/minute
- *P wave:* hidden in the preceding T wave
- *PR interval:* not visible
- *QRS complex:* 0.10 second
- *T wave:* inverted
- *QT interval:* 0.20 second
- *Other:* T-wave changes (inversion may indicate ischemia)

CAUSES

Atrial tachycardia can occur in patients with a normal heart. In those cases, it's commonly from excessive use of caffeine or other stimulants, marijuana use, electrolyte imbalance, hypoxia, or physical or psychological stress. Most commonly, however, atrial tachycardia is from an ectopic focus in the atria or primary or secondary cardiac disorders, including:

- MI
- cardiomyopathy
- congenital anomalies
- Wolff-Parkinson-White syndrome
- valvular heart disease.

This rhythm may be a component of sick sinus syndrome. Other problems resulting in atrial tachycardia include:

- cor pulmonale
- hyperthyroidism
- COPD

■ systemic hypertension
■ digoxin toxicity, the most common cause of atrial tachycardia.

CLINICAL SIGNIFICANCE

In a healthy person, nonsustained atrial tachycardia is usually benign. The increased ventricular rate that occurs in atrial tachycardia results in decreased ventricular filling time, increased myocardial oxygen consumption, and decreased oxygen supply to the myocardium. Heart failure, myocardial ischemia, and MI can result.

ECG CHARACTERISTICS

■ *Rhythm:* The atrial rhythm is usually regular. The ventricular rhythm is regular or irregular, depending on the AV conduction ratio and the type of atrial tachycardia. (See *Identifying types of atrial tachycardia.*)
■ *Rate:* The atrial rate is characterized by three or more consecutive ectopic atrial beats occurring at a rate between 150 and 250 beats/minute. The rate rarely exceeds 250 beats/minute. The ventricular rate depends on the AV conduction ratio.
■ *P wave:* The P wave may be aberrant (deviating from normal appearance) or hidden in the preceding T wave. If visible, it's usually upright and precedes each QRS complex.
■ *PR interval:* The PR interval may be unmeasurable if the P wave can't be distinguished from the preceding T wave.
■ *QRS complex:* Duration and configuration are usually normal, unless the impulses are being conducted abnormally through the ventricles.
■ *T wave:* Usually distinguishable but may be distorted by the P wave; may be inverted if ischemia is present.
■ *QT interval:* Usually within normal limits but may be shorter because of the rapid rate.

Identifying types of atrial tachycardia

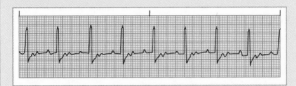

Characteristics of atrial tachycardia with block:

- *Rhythm:* atrial–regular; ventricular–regular if block is constant; irregular if block is variable
- *Rate:* atrial–140 to 250 beats/minute and a multiple of ventricular rate; ventricular–varies with block
- *P wave:* slightly abnormal; shape depends on site of ectopic pacemaker

- *PR interval:* can vary but is usually constant for conducted P waves
- *QRS complex:* usually normal
- *T wave:* usually indistinguishable
- *QT interval:* may be indiscernible
- *Other:* more than one P wave for each QRS; usually from digoxin toxicity

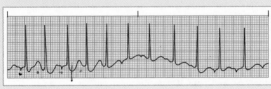

Characteristics of multifocal atrial tachycardia:

- *Rhythm:* both irregular
- *Rate:* atrial–100 to 250 beats/minute; usually under 160; ventricular–100 to 250 beats/minute
- *P wave:* configuration varying; usually at least three different P-wave shapes must appear; every P wave conducted to ventricle

- *PR interval:* varies
- *QRS complex:* usually normal; may become aberrant if arrhythmia persists
- *T wave:* usually distorted
- *QT interval:* may be indiscernible
- *Other:* none

(continued)

Identifying types of atrial tachycardia
(continued)

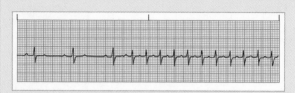

Characteristics of paroxysmal atrial tachycardia:

- *Rhythm:* atrial and ventricular rhythms may be regular or irregular and start and stop abruptly
- *Rate:* 140 to 250 beats/ minute
- *P wave:* may be inverted or retrograde; may not be visible or may be difficult to distinguish from the preceding T wave
- *PR interval:* may be unmeasurable if the P wave can't be distinguished from the preceding T wave
- *QRS complex:* can be aberrantly conducted
- *T wave:* usually indistinguishable
- *QT interval:* may be indistinguishable
- *Other:* sudden onset, typically initiated by a premature atrial contraction and sudden termination, commonly referred to as *bursts*

■ *Other:* Sometimes it may be difficult to distinguish atrial tachycardia with block from sinus arrhythmia.

SIGNS AND SYMPTOMS

The patient with atrial tachycardia will have a rapid heart rate. He may complain that his heart suddenly starts to beat faster or that he suddenly feels palpitations. Persistent tachycardia and rapid ventricular rate cause decreased cardiac output, resulting in hypotension, syncope, and dilated cardiomyopathy if left untreated.

Understanding carotid sinus massage

Carotid sinus massage may be used to interrupt paroxysmal atrial tachycardia. Massaging the carotid sinus stimulates the vagus nerve, which inhibits firing of the sinoatrial (SA) node and slows atrioventricular (AV) node conduction. As a result, the SA node can resume its function as primary pacemaker.

Carotid sinus massage involves a firm massage that lasts no longer than 5 to 10 seconds. The patient's head is turned to the left to massage the right carotid sinus, as illustrated here. Remember to never attempt simultaneous, bilateral massage.

Carotid sinus massage is contraindicated in patients with carotid bruits. Risks of the procedure include decreased heart rate, syncope, sinus arrest, increased degree of AV block, cerebral emboli, stroke, and asystole.

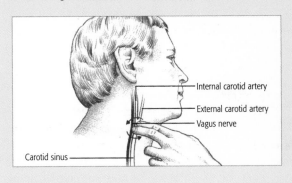

Internal carotid artery

External carotid artery

Vagus nerve

Carotid sinus

TREATMENT

Treatment depends on the type of tachycardia, the width of the QRS complex, and the stability of the patient's condition. (For specific treatments, see Tachycardia algorithm, page 264.)

The Valsalva maneuver or carotid sinus massage may be used to treat PAT. (See *Understanding carotid sinus massage*.) These maneuvers increase the parasympathetic tone, which results in a slowing of the heart rate. They also allow the SA node to resume function as the primary pacemaker.

RED FLAG Keep in mind that vagal stimulation can result in bradycardia, ventricular arrhythmias, and asystole. If vagal maneuvers are used, make sure resuscitative equipment is readily available.

LIFE STAGES Older adults may have undiagnosed carotid atherosclerosis and carotid bruits may be absent, even with significant disease. As a result, carotid sinus massage may be inappropriate in late-middle-aged and older patients.

Drug therapy (pharmacologic cardioversion) may be used to increase the degree of AV block and decrease ventricular response rate. Appropriate drugs include digoxin and beta and calcium channel blockers. When other treatments fail, or if the patient is unstable, synchronized cardioversion may be used.

Atrial overdrive pacing (also called *rapid atrial pacing* or *overdrive suppression*) may also be used to stop the arrhythmia. This technique involves suppression of spontaneous depolarization of the ectopic pacemaker by a series of paced electrical impulses at a rate slightly higher than the intrinsic ectopic atrial rate. The pacemaker cells are depolarized prematurely and, following termination of the paced electrical impulses, the SA node resumes its normal role as the pacemaker.

Radiofrequency ablation can be used to treat PAT. The ectopic focus is mapped during the electrophysiology study, and then the area is ablated. Because MAT commonly occurs in patients with COPD, the rhythm may not respond to treatment.

NURSING INTERVENTIONS

■ Monitor the patient's heart rate and rhythm.

- Assess the patient for signs and symptoms of digoxin toxicity, and monitor digoxin blood levels.
- Monitor the patient for chest pain, indications of decreased cardiac output, and signs and symptoms of heart failure or myocardial ischemia.

Atrial flutter

Atrial flutter, a supraventricular tachycardia, is characterized by a rapid atrial rate of 200 to 350 beats/minute, although it's generally around 300 beats/minute. Originating in an atrial focus, this rhythm results from a single reentry circuit in the right atria.

On an ECG, the P waves lose their normal appearance because of the rapid atrial rate. The waves blend together in a sawtooth configuration called *flutter waves,* or *F waves.* These waves are the hallmark of atrial flutter and are best seen in leads II, III, and V_1. (See *Recognizing atrial flutter,* page 104.)

CAUSES

Atrial flutter may be caused by conditions that enlarge atrial tissue and elevate atrial pressures. The arrhythmia is commonly found in patients with:

- mitral or tricuspid valvular disease
- hyperthyroidism
- pericardial disease
- digoxin toxicity
- primary myocardial disease.

The rhythm is sometimes found in patients with:

- recent cardiac surgery
- acute MI
- COPD
- systemic arterial hypoxia.

Recognizing atrial flutter

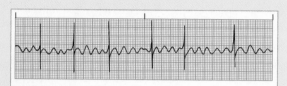

This rhythm strip illustrates atrial flutter.

- *Rhythm:* atrial–regular; ventricular–irregular
- *Rate:* atrial–280 beats/minute; ventricular–60 beats/minute
- *P wave:* classic sawtooth appearance referred to as *flutter* or *F waves*

- *PR interval:* unmeasurable
- *QRS complex:* 0.08 second
- *T wave:* unidentifiable
- *QT interval:* unmeasurable
- *Other:* atrial rate greater than ventricular rate

Atrial flutter rarely occurs in healthy people. When it does, it may indicate intrinsic cardiac disease.

CLINICAL SIGNIFICANCE

The significance of atrial flutter is determined by the number of impulses conducted through the AV node. That number is expressed as a conduction ratio, such as 2:1 or 4:1, and the resulting ventricular rate. If the ventricular rate is too slow (below 40 beats/minute) or too fast (above 150 beats/minute), cardiac output can be seriously compromised.

Usually the faster the ventricular rate, the more dangerous the arrhythmia. Rapid ventricular rates reduce ventricular filling time and coronary perfusion, which can cause angina, heart failure, pulmonary edema, hypotension, and syncope.

ECG CHARACTERISTICS

■ *Rhythm:* Atrial rhythm is regular. Ventricular rhythm depends on the AV conduction pattern; it's typically regular, although cycles may alternate. An irregular pattern may signal atrial fibrillation or indicate development of a block.

■ *Rate:* Atrial rate is 200 to 350 beats/minute. Ventricular rate depends on the degree of AV block; usually it's 60 to 100 beats/minute, but it may accelerate to 125 to 150 beats/minute.

Varying degrees of AV block produce ventricular rates that are usually one-half to one-fourth of the atrial rate. These are expressed as ratios—for example, 2:1 or 4:1. Usually, the AV node won't accept more than 180 impulses/minute and allows every second, third, or fourth impulse to be conducted. These impulses account for the ventricular rate. At the time atrial flutter is initially recognized, the ventricular response is typically above 100 beats/minute. One of the most common ventricular rates is 150 beats/minute with an atrial rate of 300, known as *2:1 block.*

■ *P wave:* Atrial flutter is characterized by abnormal P waves that produce a sawtooth appearance.

■ *PR interval:* Unmeasurable.

■ *QRS complex:* Duration is usually within normal limits, but the complex may be widened if flutter waves are buried within the complex.

■ *T wave:* Not identifiable.

■ *QT interval:* Unmeasurable because the T wave isn't identifiable.

■ *Other:* Atrial rhythm may vary between a fibrillary line and flutter waves (called *atrial fib-flutter*). At times it may be difficult to distinguish atrial flutter from atrial fibrillation.

SIGNS AND SYMPTOMS

When caring for a patient with atrial flutter, you may note that the peripheral and apical pulses are normal in rate and rhythm. That's because the pulse reflects the number of ventricular contractions, not the number of atrial impulses.

If the ventricular rate is normal, the patient may be asymptomatic. If the ventricular rate is rapid, however, the patient may experience a feeling of palpitations and may exhibit signs and symptoms of reduced cardiac output.

TREATMENT

If the patient is hemodynamically unstable, synchronized cardioversion or countershock should be given immediately. Cardioversion delivers an electrical current to the heart to correct an arrhythmia and is synchronized to discharge at the peak of the R wave. Atrial flutter is usually easily converted with a low-energy level. This causes immediate depolarization, interrupting reentry circuits and allowing the SA node to resume control as pacemaker.

The focus of treatment for hemodynamically stable patients with atrial flutter includes controlling the rate and converting the rhythm. Specific interventions depend on the patient's cardiac function, whether preexcitation syndromes are involved, and the duration (less than or greater than 48 hours) of the arrhythmia. For example, in atrial flutter with normal cardiac function and duration of rhythm less than 48 hours, direct current (DC) cardioversion may be considered; for duration greater than 48 hours, DC cardioversion wouldn't be considered because it increases the risk of thromboembolism unless the patient has been taking anticoagulants.

NURSING INTERVENTIONS

- Monitor the patient's heart rate and rhythm.
- Monitor the patient closely for signs and symptoms of low cardiac output.
- Be alert to the effects of digoxin, which depresses the SA node.
- If electrical cardioversion is indicated, prepare the patient for I.V. administration of a sedative or anesthetic as ordered. Keep resuscitative equipment at the bedside. Be alert for bradycardia because cardioversion can decrease the heart rate.

Atrial fibrillation

Atrial fibrillation, sometimes called *AFib,* is defined as chaotic, asynchronous electrical activity in atrial tissue. It's the most common arrhythmia, affecting an estimated 2 million people in the United States. It results from the firing of multiple reentry circuits in the atria. Atrial fibrillation is characterized by the absence of P waves and an irregularly irregular ventricular response.

When a number of ectopic sites in the atria initiate impulses, depolarization can't spread in an organized manner. Small sections of the atria are depolarized individually, resulting in the atrial muscle quivering instead of contracting. On an ECG, uneven baseline fibrillation waves, or f waves, appear, rather than clearly distinguishable P waves, which may be coarse or fine.

The AV node protects the ventricles from the 350 to 600 erratic atrial impulses that occur each minute by acting as a filter and blocking some of the impulses. The ventricles respond only to impulses conducted through the AV node, hence the characteristic, wide variation in R-R intervals. When the ventricular response rate drops

Recognizing atrial fibrillation

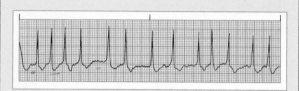

This rhythm strip illustrates atrial fibrillation.

- *Rhythm:* irregularly irregular
- *Rate:* atrial—indiscernible; ventricular—130 beats/minute
- *P wave:* absent; replaced by fine fibrillation waves, or f waves
- *PR interval:* indiscernible
- *QRS complex:* 0.08 second
- *T wave:* indiscernible
- *QT interval:* unmeasurable
- *Other:* none

below 100, atrial fibrillation is considered controlled. When the ventricular rate exceeds 100, the rhythm is considered uncontrolled. Atrial fibrillation is considered fast or uncontrolled at rates greater than 100. A "normal" ventricular response is defined as 60 to 100 beats/minute, so a ventricular rate of 100 is considered within normal.

Like atrial flutter, atrial fibrillation results in a loss of atrial kick. The rhythm may be sustained or paroxysmal, meaning that it occurs suddenly and ends abruptly. It can either be preceded by or be the result of PACs. (See *Recognizing atrial fibrillation*.)

CAUSES

Atrial fibrillation can occur after cardiothoracic surgery. Other causes of atrial fibrillation include:

- rheumatic heart disease
- valvular heart disease (especially mitral valve disease)
- hyperthyroidism

- pericarditis
- CAD
- acute MI
- hypertension
- cardiomyopathy
- atrial septal defects
- congenital heart defects
- COPD.

The rhythm may also occur in a healthy person who smokes or drinks coffee or alcohol or who's fatigued and under stress. Certain drugs, such as aminophylline and digoxin, may contribute to the development of atrial fibrillation. Endogenous catecholamine released during exercise may also trigger the arrhythmia.

CLINICAL SIGNIFICANCE

The loss of atrial kick from atrial fibrillation can result in the subsequent loss of about 20% of normal end-diastolic volume. Combined with the decreased diastolic filling time associated with a rapid heart rate, cardiac output may be reduced by 50%. In uncontrolled atrial fibrillation, the patient may develop heart failure, myocardial ischemia, or syncope.

Patients with preexisting cardiac disease, such as hypertrophic cardiomyopathy, mitral stenosis, or rheumatic heart disease, or those with prosthetic mitral valves tend to tolerate atrial fibrillation poorly and may develop severe heart failure.

RED FLAG Left untreated, atrial fibrillation can lead to cardiovascular collapse, thrombus formation, and systemic arterial or pulmonary embolism. (See Risk of restoring sinus rhythm, *page 110.)*

Risk of restoring sinus rhythm

A patient with atrial fibrillation is at increased risk for developing atrial thrombus and subsequent systemic arterial embolism. In atrial fibrillation, neither atrium contracts as a whole. As a result, blood may pool on the atrial wall, and thrombi may form. Thrombus formation places the patient at higher risk for emboli and stroke.

If normal sinus rhythm is restored and the atria contract normally, clots may break away from the atrial wall and travel through the pulmonary or systemic circulation with potentially disastrous results, such as stroke, pulmonary embolism, or arterial occlusion.

ECG CHARACTERISTICS

- *Rhythm:* Atrial and ventricular rhythms are grossly irregular, typically described as irregularly irregular.
- *Rate:* The atrial rate is indiscernible and usually exceeds 350 beats/minute. The atrial rate far exceeds the ventricular rate because most impulses aren't conducted through the AV junction. The ventricular rate usually varies from 100 to 150 beats/minute but can be below 100 beats/minute.
- *P wave:* The P wave is absent. Erratic baseline f waves appear in place of P waves. These chaotic waves represent atrial quivering from rapid atrial depolarizations.
- *PR interval:* Indiscernible.
- *QRS complex:* Duration and configuration are usually normal.
- *T wave:* Indiscernible.
- *QT interval:* Unmeasurable.
- *Other:* The patient may develop an atrial rhythm that frequently varies between coarse and fine F waves. At times, it may be difficult to distinguish atrial fibrillation from atrial flutter and MAT.

SIGNS AND SYMPTOMS

The radial pulse rate may be slower than the apical rate because the weaker contractions that occur in atrial fibrillation don't produce a palpable peripheral pulse; only the stronger ones do.

The pulse rhythm will be irregularly irregular, with a normal or abnormal heart rate. Patients with a new onset of atrial fibrillation and a rapid ventricular rate may demonstrate signs and symptoms of decreased cardiac output, including hypotension and light-headedness. Patients with chronic atrial fibrillation may be able to compensate for the decreased cardiac output and may be asymptomatic.

TREATMENT

Treatment of atrial fibrillation aims to reduce the ventricular response rate to below 100 beats/minute. This may be accomplished either by drugs that control the ventricular response or by a combination of electrical cardioversion and drug therapy, to convert the arrhythmia to normal sinus rhythm. When the onset of atrial fibrillation is acute and the patient can cooperate, vagal maneuvers or carotid sinus massage may slow the ventricular response but won't convert the arrhythmia.

If the patient is hemodynamically unstable, synchronized electrical cardioversion should be given immediately. Electrical cardioversion is most successful if used within the first 48 hours after onset and less successful the longer the duration of the arrhythmia.

RED FLAG Conversion to normal sinus rhythm will cause forceful atrial contractions to resume abruptly. If a thrombus forms in the atria, the resumption of contractions can result in systemic emboli. (See How synchronized cardioversion works, *page 112.)*

How synchronized cardioversion works

A patient experiencing an arrhythmia that leads to reduced cardiac output may be a candidate for synchronized cardioversion. This procedure may be done electively or as an emergency. For instance, it may be used electively in a patient with recurrent atrial fibrillation or urgently in a patient with ventricular tachycardia and a pulse.

Synchronized cardioversion is similar to defibrillation, also called *unsynchronized cardioversion.* Synchronizing the energy delivered to the patient reduces the risk that the current will strike during the relative refractory period of a cardiac cycle and induce ventricular fibrillation (VF). This vulnerable period occurs early in the T wave.

In synchronized cardioversion, the R wave on the patient's ECG is synchronized with the cardioverter (defibrillator). After the firing buttons have been pressed, the cardioverter discharges energy when it senses the next R wave.

Keep in mind that a slight delay occurs between the time the discharge buttons are depressed and the moment the energy is actually discharged. When using handheld paddles, continue to hold the paddles on the patient's chest until the energy is delivered.

Remember to reset the SYNC MODE on the defibrillator after each synchronized cardioversion. Resetting this switch is necessary because most defibrillators will automatically reset to an unsynchronized mode.

If VF occurs during the procedure, turn off the SYNC button and immediately deliver an unsynchronized defibrillation to terminate the arrhythmia. Be aware that synchronized cardioversion carries the risk of lethal arrhythmia when used in patients with digoxin toxicity.

The focus of treatment for hemodynamically stable patients with atrial fibrillation includes controlling the rate, converting the rhythm, and providing anticoagulation if indicated. Specific interventions depend on the patient's cardiac function, whether preexcitation syndromes are involved, and the duration of the arrhythmia.

Drugs to control the ventricular response rate include digoxin and beta and calcium channel blockers. When the rhythm is converted to a normal sinus rhythm, antiarrhythmics, such as amiodarone, quinidine, sotalol, and propafenone, are used to maintain the rhythm. Some of these drugs prolong the atrial refractory period, giving the SA node an opportunity to reestablish its role as the heart's pacemaker. Others primarily slow AV node conduction, controlling the ventricular response rate. Nonpharmacologic treatment may include atrial pacing or radiofrequency ablation.

NURSING INTERVENTIONS

■ Monitor the patient's heart rate and rhythm.
■ Assess the peripheral and apical pulses. If the patient isn't on a cardiac monitor, be alert for an irregular pulse and differences in the radial and apical pulse rates.
■ Assess for symptoms of decreased cardiac output and heart failure.
■ If drug therapy is used, monitor drug levels and observe the patient for evidence of toxicity.
■ Tell the patient to report pulse rate changes, syncope or dizziness, chest pain, and signs of heart failure, such as dyspnea and peripheral edema.

Ashman's phenomenon

Ashman's phenomenon refers to the aberrant conduction of premature supraventricular beats to the ventricles. (See *Recognizing Ashman's phenomenon,* page 114.) This benign phenomenon is frequently associated with atrial fibrillation but can occur with any arrhythmia that affects the R-R interval.

Recognizing Ashman's phenomenon

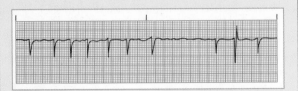

This rhythm strip illustrates Ashman's phenomenon.

- *Rhythm:* atrial and ventricular—irregular
- *Rate:* underlying rhythm of 90 beats/minute
- *P wave:* absent; fibrillation waves
- *PR interval:* unmeasurable

- *QRS complex:* 0.12 second; right bundle-branch block pattern present on Ashman beat
- *T wave:* deflection opposite that of QRS complex in the Ashman beat
- *QT interval:* unmeasurable
- *Other:* no compensatory pause after the aberrant beat

CAUSES

Ashman's phenomenon is caused by intermittent bundle-branch block resulting from beat-by-beat loss of conduction. In theory, a conduction aberration occurs when a short cycle follows a long cycle because the refractory period varies with the length of the cycle. An impulse that ends a short cycle preceded by a long one is more likely to reach refractory tissue.

The normal refractory period for the right bundle branch is slightly longer than the left one, so premature beats frequently reach the right bundle when it's partially or completely refractory. Because of this tendency, the abnormal beat is usually seen as a right bundle-branch block (RBBB).

CLINICAL SIGNIFICANCE

The importance of recognizing aberrantly conducted beats is primarily to prevent misdiagnosis and subsequent mistaken treatment of ventricular ectopy.

ECG CHARACTERISTICS

■ *Rhythm:* Atrial and ventricular rhythms are irregular.
■ *Rate:* Atrial and ventricular rates reflect the underlying rhythm.
■ *P wave:* The P wave has an abnormal configuration. It may be visible. If present in the underlying rhythm, the P wave is unchanged.
■ *PR interval:* If measurable, the interval commonly changes on the premature beat.
■ *QRS complex:* Configuration is usually altered, revealing an RBBB pattern.
■ *T wave:* Deflection opposite that of the QRS complex occurs in most leads as a result of RBBB.
■ *QT interval:* Usually has changed as a result of the RBBB.
■ *Other:* There's no compensatory pause after an aberrant beat. The aberrancy may continue for several beats and typically ends a short cycle preceded by a long cycle.

SIGNS AND SYMPTOMS

No signs and symptoms are found in this phenomenon.

TREATMENT

No treatment is necessary, but treatment may be required for accompanying arrhythmias.

NURSING INTERVENTIONS

■ Monitor the patient's heart rate and rhythm.

Recognizing wandering pacemaker

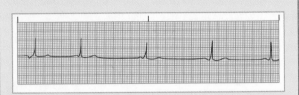

This rhythm strip illustrates wandering pacemaker.

- *Rhythm:* atrial and ventricular—irregular
- *Rate:* atrial and ventricular—50 beats/minute
- *P wave:* changes in size and shape; first P wave inverted, second upright
- *PR interval:* varied
- *QRS complex:* 0.08 second
- *T wave:* normal
- *QT interval:* 0.44 second
- *Other:* none

Wandering pacemaker

Wandering pacemaker, also called *wandering atrial pacemaker,* is an atrial arrhythmia that results when the site of impulse formation shifts from the SA node to another area above the ventricles. The origin of the impulse may wander beat to beat from the SA node to ectopic sites in the atria, or to the AV junctional tissue. The P wave and PR interval vary from beat to beat as the pacemaker site changes. (See *Recognizing wandering pacemaker.*)

CAUSES

In most cases, wandering pacemaker is caused by increased parasympathetic (vagal) influences on the SA node or AV junction. It can also be caused by COPD, valvular heart disease, digoxin toxicity, and inflammation of the atrial tissue.

CLINICAL SIGNIFICANCE

The arrhythmia may be normal in young patients and is common in athletes who have slow heart rates. The arrhythmia may be difficult to identify because it's commonly transient. Although wandering pacemaker is rarely serious, chronic arrhythmias are a sign of heart disease and should be monitored.

ECG CHARACTERISTICS

■ *Rhythm:* The atrial rhythm varies slightly, with an irregular P-P interval. The ventricular rhythm varies slightly, with an irregular R-R interval.

■ *Rate:* Atrial and ventricular rates vary but are usually within normal limits, or below 60 beats/minute.

■ *P wave:* Altered size and configuration are due to the changing pacemaker site. The P wave may also be absent or inverted or may follow the QRS complex if the impulse originates in the AV junction. A combination of these variations may appear.

■ *PR interval:* The PR interval varies from beat to beat as the pacemaker site changes but usually less than 0.20 second. If the impulse originates in the AV junction, the PR interval will be less than 0.12 second. This variation in PR interval will cause a slightly irregular R-R interval. When the P wave is present, the PR interval may be normal or shortened.

■ *QRS complex:* Ventricular depolarization is normal, so duration of the QRS complex is usually within normal limits and is of normal configuration.

■ *T wave:* Normal size and configuration.

■ *QT interval:* Usually within normal limits but may vary.

■ *Other:* At times, it may be difficult to distinguish wandering pacemaker from PACs.

SIGNS AND SYMPTOMS

Patients are generally asymptomatic and unaware of the arrhythmia. The pulse rate may be normal or below 60 beats/minute, and the rhythm may be regular or slightly irregular.

TREATMENT

Usually, no treatment is needed for asymptomatic patients. If the patient is symptomatic, however, his drugs should be reviewed and the underlying cause investigated and treated.

NURSING INTERVENTIONS

■ Monitor the patient's heart rate and rhythm.
■ Watch for signs of hemodynamic instability, such as hypotension and changes in mental status.

5

JUNCTIONAL ARRHYTHMIAS

Junctional arrhythmias originate in the atrioventricular (AV) junction—the area in and around the AV node and the bundle of His. The specialized pacemaker cells in the AV junction take over as the heart's pacemaker if the sinoatrial (SA) node doesn't function properly or if the electrical impulses originating in the SA node are blocked. These junctional pacemaker cells have an inherent firing rate of 40 to 60 beats/minute.

In normal impulse conduction, the AV node slows transmission of the impulse from the atria to the ventricles, which allows the ventricles to fill as much as possible before they contract. However, these impulses don't always follow the normal conduction pathway. (See *Conduction in Wolff-Parkinson-White syndrome,* page 120.)

Because of the location of the AV junction within the conduction pathway, electrical impulses originating in this area cause abnormal depolarization of the heart. The impulse is conducted retrograde (backward) to depolarize the atria and antegrade (forward) to depolarize the ventricles.

Depolarization of the atria can precede depolarization of the ventricles, or the ventricles can be depolarized before the atria. Depolarization of the atria and ventricles

Conduction in Wolff-Parkinson-White syndrome

Electrical impulses in the heart don't always follow normal conduction pathways. In pre-excitation syndromes, electrical impulses enter the ventricles from the atria through an accessory pathway that bypasses the atrioventricular junction. Wolff-Parkinson-White (WPW) syndrome is a common type of preexcitation syndrome.

WPW syndrome commonly occurs in young children and in adults ages 20 to 35. The syndrome causes the PR interval to shorten and the QRS complex to lengthen as a result of a delta wave. Delta waves, which are a slurring of the upstroke of a QRS complex, are produced as a result of the premature depolarization or preexcitation of a portion of the ventricles.

WPW is clinically significant because the accessory pathway—in this case, Kent's bundle—may result in paroxysmal tachyarrhythmias by reentry and rapid conduction mechanisms.

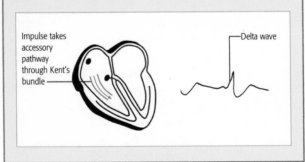

Impulse takes accessory pathway through Kent's bundle

Delta wave

can also occur simultaneously. (See *Locating the P wave.*) Retrograde depolarization of the atria results in inverted P waves in leads II, III, and aV$_F$, which are leads in which you would normally see upright P waves.

Remember that arrhythmias causing inverted P waves on an electrocardiogram (ECG) may originate in the atria

Locating the P wave

When the specialized pacemaker cells in the atrioventricular junction take over as the dominant pacemaker of the heart:
● depolarization of the atria can precede depolarization of the ventricles
● the ventricles can be depolarized before the atria
● simultaneous depolarization of the atria and ventricles can occur.

   The rhythm strips shown here demonstrate the various locations of the P waves in junctional arrhythmias, depending on the direction of depolarization.

INVERTED P WAVE	**INVERTED P WAVE**	**INVERTED P WAVE** (HIDDEN)
If the atria are depolarized first, the P wave will occur before the QRS complex.	If the ventricles are depolarized first, the P wave will occur after the QRS complex.	If the ventricles and atria are depolarized simultaneously, the P wave will be hidden in the QRS complex.

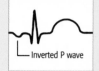

Inverted P wave

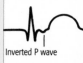

Inverted P wave

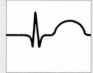

or AV junction. Atrial arrhythmias are sometimes mistaken for junctional arrhythmias because impulses are generated so low in the atria that they cause retrograde depolarization and inverted P waves.

Looking at the PR interval will help you determine whether an arrhythmia is atrial or junctional. An arrhythmia with:
■ an inverted P wave and with a normal PR interval (0.12 to 0.20 second) originates in the atria.

■ a PR interval less than 0.12 second originates in the AV junction.

Premature junctional contractions

A premature junctional contraction (PJC) is a junctional beat that occurs before a normal sinus beat and causes an irregular rhythm. These ectopic beats commonly occur as a result of enhanced automaticity in the junctional tissue or bundle of His. As with all impulses generated in the AV junction, the atria are depolarized retrograde, causing an inverted P wave. The ventricles are depolarized normally. (See *Recognizing a premature junctional contraction.*)

CAUSES
PJCs may be caused by:
■ digoxin toxicity
■ excessive caffeine intake
■ amphetamine ingestion
■ alcohol use
■ stress
■ coronary artery disease
■ myocardial ischemia
■ inferior wall myocardial infarction (MI)
■ valvular heart disease
■ valvular disease
■ pericarditis
■ heart failure
■ chronic pulmonary disease
■ hyperthyroidism
■ electrolyte imbalances
■ inflammatory changes in the AV junction following heart surgery.

Recognizing a premature junctional contraction

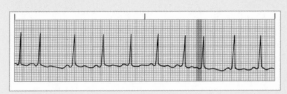

This rhythm strip illustrates sinus rhythm with premature junctional contractions (PJCs).

- *Rhythm:* irregular atrial and ventricular rhythms during PJCs
- *Rate:* 100 beats/minute
- *P wave:* inverted and precedes the QRS complex (see shaded area)
- *PR interval:* 0.14 second for the underlying rhythm and 0.06 second for the PJC
- *QRS complex:* 0.06 second
- *T wave:* normal configuration
- *QT interval:* 0.36 second
- *Other:* noncompensatory pause

CLINICAL SIGNIFICANCE

PJCs are generally considered harmless.

RED FLAG Frequent PJCs indicate junctional irritability and can precipitate a more serious arrhythmia such as junctional tachycardia. In patients taking digoxin, PJCs are a common early sign of toxicity.

ECG CHARACTERISTICS

- *Rhythm:* Atrial and ventricular rhythms are irregular during PJCs; the underlying rhythm may be regular.
- *Rate:* Atrial and ventricular rates reflect the underlying rhythm.
- *P wave:* The P wave is usually inverted. It may occur before or after the QRS complex, be absent, or be hid-

den in the QRS complex. Look for an inverted P wave in leads II, III, and aV$_F$. Depending on the initial direction of depolarization, the P wave may fall before, during, or after the QRS complex.

■ *PR interval:* If the P wave precedes the QRS complex, the PR interval is shortened (less than 0.12 second); otherwise, it can't be measured.

■ *QRS complex:* Because the ventricles are usually depolarized normally, the QRS complex usually has a normal configuration and a normal duration of less than 0.12 second.

■ *T wave:* Usually normal configuration.

■ *QT interval:* Usually within normal limits.

■ *Other:* A noncompensatory pause reflecting retrograde atrial conduction commonly accompanies PJCs.

SIGNS AND SYMPTOMS

The patient is usually asymptomatic. He may complain of palpitations or a feeling of "skipped beats." You may be able to palpate an irregular pulse when PJCs occur. If PJCs are frequent enough, the patient may experience hypotension from a transient decrease in cardiac output.

TREATMENT

PJCs usually don't require treatment unless the patient is symptomatic. In those cases, the underlying cause should be treated. For example, in digoxin toxicity, the drug should be stopped and drug level monitored. If ectopic beats occur because of caffeine, the patient should decrease or eliminate his caffeine intake.

NURSING INTERVENTIONS

■ Monitor heart rate and rhythm.

■ Monitor the patient for hemodynamic instability.

Junctional escape rhythm

A junctional escape rhythm, also referred to as *junctional rhythm,* is an arrhythmia originating in the AV junction. In this arrhythmia, the AV junction takes over as a secondary, or escape, pacemaker. This usually occurs only when a higher pacemaker site in the atria, typically the SA node, fails as the heart's dominant pacemaker.

Remember that the AV junction can take over as the heart's dominant pacemaker if:

■ the firing rate of the higher pacemaker sites falls below the AV junction firing rate or fails to generate an impulse
■ the conduction of the impulses is blocked.

RED FLAG Because junctional escape beats prevent ventricular standstill, they should never be suppressed.

In a junctional escape rhythm, as in all junctional arrhythmias, the atria are depolarized by means of retrograde conduction. The P waves are inverted, and impulse conduction through the ventricles is normal. The normal intrinsic firing rate for cells in the AV junction is 40 to 60 beats/minute. (See *Recognizing junctional escape rhythm,* page 126.)

LIFE STAGES Junctional escape beats may occur in healthy children during sleep. They may also occur in healthy athletic adults. In these situations, no treatment is necessary.

CAUSES

This rhythm can be caused by any condition that disturbs normal SA node function or impulse conduction. Causes of the arrhythmia include:

■ SA node ischemia
■ hypoxia
■ electrolyte imbalances

Recognizing junctional escape rhythm

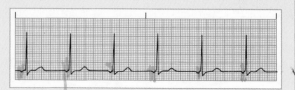

This rhythm strip illustrates junctional escape rhythm.

- *Rhythm:* regular
- *Rate:* 60 beats/minute
- *P wave:* inverted and preceding each QRS complex
- *PR interval:* 0.10 second
- *QRS complex:* 0.10 second
- *T wave:* normal
- *QT interval:* 0.44 second
- *Other:* none

- valvular heart disease
- heart failure
- cardiomyopathy
- myocarditis
- sick sinus syndrome
- increased parasympathetic (vagal) tone.

Drugs, such as digoxin, calcium channel blockers, and beta blockers, can also cause a junctional escape rhythm.

CLINICAL SIGNIFICANCE

The clinical significance depends on how well the patient tolerates a decreased heart rate (40 to 60 beats/minute) and an associated decrease in cardiac output. In addition to a decreased cardiac output from a slower heart rate, depolarization of the atria either after or simultaneously with ventricular depolarization results in loss of atrial kick. Remember that junctional escape rhythms protect the heart from life-threatening ventricular escape rhythms.

ECG CHARACTERISTICS

■ *Rhythm:* Atrial and ventricular rhythms are regular.
■ *Rate:* The atrial and ventricular rates are 40 to 60 beats/minute.
■ *P wave:* The P wave is usually inverted (look for inverted P waves in leads II, III, and aV$_F$). The P wave may occur before or after the QRS complex, be hidden within it, or may be absent.
■ *PR interval:* If the P wave precedes the QRS complex, the PR interval is shortened (less than 0.12 second); otherwise, it can't be measured.
■ *QRS complex:* Duration is usually within normal limits; configuration is usually normal.
■ *T wave:* Usually normal configuration.
■ *QT interval:* Usually within normal limits.
■ *Other:* None.

SIGNS AND SYMPTOMS

The patient will have a slow, regular pulse rate of 40 to 60 beats/minute. The patient may be asymptomatic.

RED FLAG Pulse rates below 60 beats/minute may lead to inadequate cardiac output, causing hypotension, syncope, or blurred vision.

TREATMENT

Treatment involves identification and correction of the underlying cause, whenever possible. (For specific treatments, see the Bradycardia algorithm, pages 260 and 261.) Atropine may be used to increase the heart rate while waiting for a temporary or permanent pacemaker to be inserted.

NURSING INTERVENTIONS

- ■ Monitor heart rate and rhythm.
- ■ Monitor the patient's digoxin and electrolyte levels.
- ■ Watch for signs of decreased cardiac output, such as hypotension, syncope, and blurred vision.

Accelerated junctional rhythm ✓

An accelerated junctional rhythm is an arrhythmia that originates in the AV junction and is usually caused by enhanced automaticity of the AV junctional tissue. It's called accelerated because it occurs at a rate of 60 to 100 beats/minute, exceeding the inherent junctional escape rate of 40 to 60 beats/minute.

Because the rate is below 100 beats/minute, the arrhythmia isn't classified as junctional tachycardia. The atria are depolarized by means of retrograde conduction, and the ventricles are depolarized normally. (See *Recognizing accelerated junctional rhythm.*)

CAUSES

Digoxin toxicity is a common cause. Other causes include:

- ■ electrolyte disturbances
- ■ valvular heart disease
- ■ rheumatic heart disease
- ■ heart failure
- ■ myocarditis
- ■ cardiac surgery
- ■ inferior- or posterior-wall MI.

CLINICAL SIGNIFICANCE

Patients are generally asymptomatic because the rate corresponds to the normal inherent firing rate of the SA node (60 to 100 beats/minute). However, symptoms of de-

Recognizing accelerated junctional rhythm

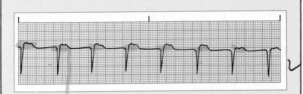

This rhythm strip illustrates accelerated junctional rhythm.

- *Rhythm:* regular ✓
- *Rate:* 80 beats/minute ✓
- *P wave:* absent ✓
- *PR interval:* unmeasurable
- *QRS complex:* 0.10 second ✓
- *T wave:* normal
- *QT interval:* 0.32 second ✓
- *Other:* none

creased cardiac output, including hypotension and syncope, can occur if atrial depolarization occurs after or simultaneously with ventricular depolarization, which causes the subsequent loss of atrial kick.

ECG CHARACTERISTICS

- *Rhythm:* Atrial and ventricular rhythms are regular.
- *Rate:* Atrial and ventricular rates range from 60 to 100 beats/minute.
- *P wave:* If the P wave is present, it will be inverted in leads II, III, and aV_F. It may proceed, follow, or be hidden in the QRS complex or be absent entirely.
- *PR interval:* If the P wave occurs before the QRS complex, the PR interval is shortened (less than 0.12 second). Otherwise, it can't be measured.
- *QRS complex:* Duration is usually within normal limits, though it may be slightly prolonged. Configuration is usually normal.
- *T wave:* Usually within normal limits.

■ *QT interval:* Usually within normal limits.
■ *Other:* None.

⏱ **LIFE STAGES** *Until age 3, the AV nodal escape rhythm is 50 to 80 beats/minute. Consequently, a junctional rhythm is considered accelerated in infants and toddlers only when greater than 80 beats/minute.*

SIGNS AND SYMPTOMS

The pulse rate will be normal with a regular rhythm. The patient may be asymptomatic because accelerated junctional rhythm has the same rate as sinus rhythm. However, if cardiac output is decreased, the patient may exhibit symptoms, such as hypotension, changes in mental status, and weak peripheral pulses.

TREATMENT

Treatment involves identifying and correcting the underlying cause.

NURSING INTERVENTIONS

■ Monitor heart rate and rhythm.
■ Watch for evidence of decreased cardiac output and hemodynamic instability.
■ Monitor serum digoxin and electrolyte levels.

Junctional tachycardia

In junctional tachycardia, three or more premature junctional contractions occur in a row. This supraventricular tachycardia generally occurs as a result of enhanced automaticity of the AV junction, which causes the AV junction to override the SA node as the dominant pacemaker.

In junctional tachycardia, the atria are depolarized by retrograde conduction. Conduction through the ventricles

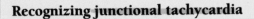

Recognizing junctional tachycardia

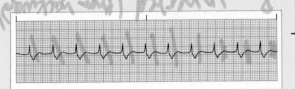

This rhythm strip illustrates junctional tachycardia.

- *Rhythm:* atrial and ventricular—regular
- *Rate:* atrial and ventricular—110 beats/minute
- *P wave:* inverted; follows QRS complex
- *PR interval:* unmeasurable
- *QRS complex:* 0.08 second
- *T wave:* normal
- *QT interval:* 0.36 second
- *Other:* none

is normal. The rate is usually 100 to 200 beats/minute. (See *Recognizing junctional tachycardia.*)

CAUSES

Digoxin toxicity is the most common cause. In such cases, the arrhythmia can be aggravated by hypokalemia. Other causes of junctional tachycardia include:

- inferior- or posterior-wall infarction or ischemia
- inflammation of the AV junction following heart surgery
- heart failure
- electrolyte imbalances
- valvular heart disease
- congenital heart disease in children.

CLINICAL SIGNIFICANCE

The clinical significance depends on the rate and underlying cause. At higher ventricular rates, junctional tachycardia may reduce cardiac output by decreasing ventricular filling time. A loss of atrial kick also occurs with atrial depolarization that follows or occurs simultaneously with ventricular depolarization.

ECG CHARACTERISTICS

- *Rhythm:* Atrial and ventricular rhythms are usually regular. The atrial rhythm may be difficult to determine if the P wave is absent or hidden in the QRS complex or preceding T wave.
- *Rate:* Atrial and ventricular rates exceed 100 beats/minute (usually between 100 and 200 beats/minute). The atrial rate may be difficult to determine if the P wave is absent or hidden in the QRS complex or the preceding T wave.
- *P wave:* The P wave is usually inverted in leads II, III, and aV$_F$. The P wave may occur before or after the QRS complex, be hidden in the QRS complex, or be absent.
- *PR interval:* If the P wave precedes the QRS complex, the PR interval is shortened (less than 0.12 second); otherwise, the PR interval can't be measured.
- *QRS complex:* Duration is within normal limits; configuration is usually normal.
- *T wave:* Configuration is usually normal but may be abnormal if the P wave is hidden in the T wave. The fast rate may make T waves indiscernible.
- *QT interval:* Usually within normal limits.
- *Other:* None.

SIGNS AND SYMPTOMS

The patient's pulse rate will be above 100 beats/minute and have a regular rhythm.

RED FLAG *Patients with a rapid heart rate may experience signs and symptoms of decreased cardiac output and hemodynamic instability including hypotension.*

TREATMENT

The underlying cause should be identified and treated. If the cause is digoxin toxicity, the drug should be stopped. Digoxin may be used if it isn't the cause of the tachycardia. Patients with recurrent junctional tachycardia may be treated with ablation therapy, followed by permanent pacemaker insertion.

If symptomatic with paroxysmal onset of junctional tachycardia, vagal maneuvers and drugs such as adenosine may slow the heart rate. If the patient has normal heart function, beta blockers, calcium channel blockers, or amiodarone may be given.

NURSING INTERVENTIONS

■ Monitor heart rate and rhythm.
■ Watch for signs of decreased cardiac output.
■ Watch for evidence of digoxin toxicity and monitor digoxin level.

6

VENTRICULAR ARRHYTHMIAS

Ventricular arrhythmias originate in the ventricles below the bifurcation of the bundle of His. These arrhythmias occur when electrical impulses depolarize the myocardium using a pathway different from normal impulse conduction.

Ventricular arrhythmias appear on an electrocardiogram (ECG) in characteristic ways. The QRS complex in most of these arrhythmias is wider than normal because of the prolonged conduction time through, and abnormal depolarization of, the ventricles. The deflections of the T wave and the QRS complex are in opposite directions because ventricular repolarization, as well as ventricular depolarization, is abnormal. The P wave in many ventricular arrhythmias is absent because atrial depolarization doesn't occur. If a P wave is present, it originates in the sinus node, causing it to be dissociated from the ventricular rhythm.

When electrical impulses come from the ventricles instead of the atria, atrial kick is lost and cardiac output can decrease by as much as 30%. As a result, patients with ventricular arrhythmias may show signs and symptoms of decreased cardiac output, including:

- hypotension
- angina

■ syncope
■ respiratory distress.

Although ventricular arrhythmias may be benign, they may also be serious because the ventricles are ultimately responsible for cardiac output. Rapid recognition and treatment of ventricular arrhythmias increase the chances of successful return to normal rhythm.

Premature ventricular contractions

Premature ventricular contractions (PVCs) are ectopic beats that originate in the ventricles and occur earlier than expected. PVCs may occur in healthy people without being clinically significant.

However, when PVCs occur in patients with underlying heart disease, they may herald the development of lethal ventricular arrhythmias, including ventricular tachycardia (VT) and ventricular fibrillation (VF).

PVCs may occur singly, in pairs (couplets), or in clusters. PVCs may also appear in patterns, such as bigeminy or trigeminy. (See *Recognizing premature ventricular contractions,* page 136.) In many cases, PVCs are followed by a compensatory pause because the timing from the sinoatrial (SA) node isn't interrupted. PVCs may be uniform in appearance, arising from a single ectopic ventricular pacemaker site, or multiform, with QRS complexes that differ in size, shape, and direction, indicating a different pattern of ventricular depolarization.

PVCs may also be described as unifocal or multifocal. Unifocal PVCs originate from the same ventricular ectopic pacemaker site, whereas multifocal PVCs originate from different ectopic pacemaker sites in the ventricles.

Recognizing premature ventricular contractions

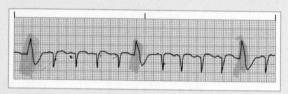

This rhythm strip illustrates normal sinus rhythm with premature ventricular contractions (PVCs).

- *Rhythm:* irregular
- *Rate:* 120 beats/minute
- *P wave:* none with PVC, but P wave present with other QRS complexes
- *PR interval:* 0.12 second in underlying rhythm
- *QRS complex:* early, with bizarre configuration and duration of 0.14 second in PVC;

QRS complexes are 0.08 second in underlying rhythm
- *T wave:* normal; opposite direction from QRS complex in PVC
- *QT interval:* 0.28 second with underlying rhythm
- *Other:* compensatory pause after PVC

CAUSES

PVCs may be caused by enhanced or abnormal automaticity in the ventricular conduction system or muscle tissue. The irritable focus results from a disruption of the normal electrolyte shifts during cellular depolarization and repolarization. Possible causes of PVCs include:

- caffeine or alcohol ingestion
- drug intoxication, particularly with cocaine, amphetamines, and tricyclic antidepressants
- electrolyte imbalances, such as hypokalemia, hyperkalemia, hypomagnesemia, and hypocalcemia
- enlargement or hypertrophy of the ventricular chambers

- hypoxia
- increased sympathetic stimulation
- irritation of the ventricles by pacemaker electrodes or a pulmonary artery catheter
- metabolic acidosis
- myocardial ischemia and infarction
- myocarditis
- proarrhythmic effects of some antiarrhythmics
- sympathomimetics, such as epinephrine and isoproterenol
- tobacco use.

CLINICAL SIGNIFICANCE

PVCs are significant for two reasons. First, they can lead to more serious arrhythmias, such as VT or VF. The risk of developing a more serious arrhythmia increases in patients with ischemic or damaged hearts or with significant electrolyte imbalance.

PVCs also decrease cardiac output, especially if ectopic beats are frequent or repetitive. The decrease in cardiac output with a PVC stems from reduced ventricular diastolic filling time and the loss of atrial kick for that beat. The clinical impact of PVCs hinges on the body's ability to maintain adequate perfusion and the duration of the abnormal rhythm.

To help determine the seriousness of PVCs, ask yourself these questions:

- How often do they occur? In patients with chronic PVCs, an increase in frequency or a change in the pattern of PVCs from the baseline rhythm may signal a more serious condition.
- What's the pattern of PVCs? If the ECG shows a dangerous pattern—such as paired PVCs, PVCs with more than one focus, a bigeminal rhythm, or R-on-T phenomenon (when a PVC strikes on the down slope of

Patterns of potentially dangerous premature ventricular contractions

Some premature ventricular contractions (PVCs) are more dangerous than others. Here are examples of patterns of potentially dangerous PVCs.

PAIRED PVCS

Two PVCs in a row, called *paired PVCs* or a *ventricular couplet* (see shaded areas), can produce ventricular tachycardia (VT). That's because the second contraction usually indicates the presence of a reentry circuit. A burst, or a salvo, of three or more PVCs in a row is considered a run of VT.

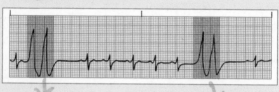

MULTIFORM PVCS

Multiform PVCs, which look different from one another, arise from different sites or from the same site with abnormal conduction. (See shaded areas.) Multiform PVCs may indicate severe heart disease or digoxin toxicity.

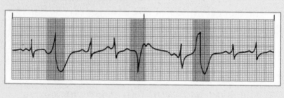

the preceding normal T wave)—the patient may require immediate treatment. (See *Patterns of potentially dangerous premature ventricular contractions.*)

■ Are they really PVCs? Make sure the complex is a PVC, not another, less dangerous arrhythmia. PVCs may be

Patterns of potentially dangerous premature ventricular contractions *(continued)*

BIGEMINY AND TRIGEMINY

PVCs that occur every other beat (bigeminy) or every third beat (trigeminy) indicate increased irritability and may lead to VT or ventricular fibrillation. (See shaded areas.) The rhythm strip shown below illustrates ventricular bigeminy.

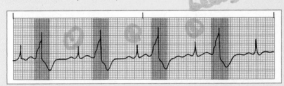

R-ON-T PHENOMENON

In R-on-T phenomenon, a PVC occurs so early that it falls on the T wave of the preceding beat (See shaded area.) Because the cells haven't fully repolarized, VT or VF can result.

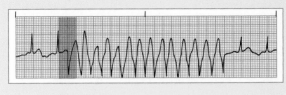

mistaken for ventricular escape beats or normal impulses with aberrant ventricular conduction. Ventricular escape beats serve as a safety mechanism to protect the heart from ventricular standstill. Some supraventricular impulses may follow an abnormal conduction pathway causing an abnormal appearance to the QRS complex. In any event, never delay treatment if the patient is unstable.

ECG CHARACTERISTICS

■ *Rhythm:* Atrial and ventricular rhythms are irregular during PVCs; the underlying rhythm may be regular.

■ *Rate:* Atrial and ventricular rates reflect the underlying rhythm.

■ *P wave:* Usually absent in the ectopic beat, but with retrograde conduction to the atria, the P wave may appear after the QRS complex. It's usually normal if present in the underlying rhythm.

■ *PR interval:* Unmeasurable except in the underlying rhythm.

■ *QRS complex:* Occurrence is earlier than expected. Duration exceeds 0.12 second, and is usually longer than 0.16 second with a bizarre and wide configuration. Configuration of the QRS complex is usually normal in the underlying rhythm.

■ *T wave:* Occurrence is in opposite direction to QRS complex. When a PVC strikes on the down slope of the preceding normal T wave—the R-on-T phenomenon—it can trigger more serious rhythm disturbances.

■ *QT interval:* Not usually measured, except in the underlying rhythm.

■ *Other:* A PVC may be followed by a compensatory pause, which can be full or incomplete. The sum of a full compensatory pause and the preceding R-R interval is equal to the sum of two R-R intervals of the underlying rhythm. If the SA node is depolarized by the PVC, the timing of the SA node is reset, and the compensatory pause is called incomplete. In this case, the sum of an incomplete compensatory pause and the preceding R-R interval is less than the sum of two R-R intervals of the underlying rhythm. A PVC occurring between two normally conducted QRS complexes without greatly disturbing the underlying rhythm is referred to as inter-

polated. A full compensatory pause, usually accompanying PVCs, is absent with interpolated PVCs.

Sometimes it's difficult to distinguish PVCs from aberrant ventricular conduction. (See *Distinguishing premature
ventricular contractions from ventricular aberrancy,* pages
142 and 143.)

SIGNS AND SYMPTOMS

A patient with PVCs usually has a pulse rate within the
normal range of 60 to 100 beats/minute. When a PVC occurs, the pulse rhythm will be momentarily irregular.

With PVCs, the patient will have a weaker pulse wave
after the premature beat and a longer-than-normal pause
between pulse waves. At times, you may not be able to
palpate a pulse after the PVC. If the carotid pulse is visible,
however, you may see a weaker arterial wave after the premature beat. When auscultating for heart sounds, you'll
hear an abnormally early heart sound with each PVC.

A patient with PVCs may be asymptomatic. However,
patients with frequent PVCs may complain of palpitations.
The patient may also exhibit signs and symptoms of decreased cardiac output, including hypotension and syncope.

TREATMENT

If the PVCs are infrequent and the patient has normal
heart function and is asymptomatic, the arrhythmia probably won't require treatment. If symptoms or a dangerous
form of PVCs occur, the type of treatment given will depend on the cause of the problem.

If PVCs have a purely cardiac origin, drugs to suppress
ventricular irritability may be used. Procainamide, amiodarone, and lidocaine are typically used. When PVCs have
a noncardiac origin, treatment is aimed at correcting the
cause. For example, drug therapy may be adjusted or the
patient's acidosis or electrolyte imbalance corrected.

Distinguishing premature ventricular contractions from ventricular aberrancy

Perhaps one of the most challenging look-alikes—premature ventricular contractions (PVCs) versus ventricular aberrancy—can sometimes be distinguished with complete confidence only in the electrophysiology laboratory. Ventricular aberrancy, or aberrant ventricular conduction, occurs when an electrical impulse originating in the sinoatrial node, atria, or atrioventricular junction is temporarily conducted abnormally through the bundle branches.

The abnormal conduction results in a bundle-branch block and usually stems from the arrival of electrical impulses at the bundle branches before the branches have been sufficiently repolarized.

To distinguish between PVCs and ventricular aberrancy, examine the deflection of the QRS complex in lead V_1. Determine whether the QRS complex is primarily positive or negative. Based on this information, follow these clues to guide your analysis.

MOSTLY POSITIVE QRS

• Right bundle-branch aberrancy will have a triphasic rSR' configuration in V_1 and a triphasic qRS configuration in V_6.

• If there are two positive peaks in V_1 and the left peak is taller, the beat is probably a PVC.

• PVCs will be monophasic or biphasic in V_1, and biphasic in V_6, with a deep S wave.

COMPARING PVC WITH RIGHT BUNDLE-BRANCH ABERRANCY

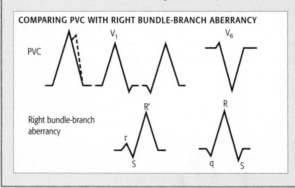

Distinguishing premature ventricular contractions from ventricular aberrancy
(continued)

MOSTLY NEGATIVE QRS

● Left bundle-branch aberrancy will have a narrow R wave with a quick downstroke in leads V_1 and V_2, and no Q wave in V_6.

● PVCs will have an R wave (longer than 0.03 second) and a notched or slurred S-wave downstroke in leads V_1 and V_2, with a duration of more than 0.06 second from the onset of the R wave to the deepest point of the S wave in V_1 and V_2, and a Q wave in V_6.

● P waves commonly precede aberrancies. P waves don't generally precede PVCs.

● Aberrancies usually have a QRS duration of 0.12 to 0.14 second. PVCs are more likely to have a QRS duration of 0.16 second or more.

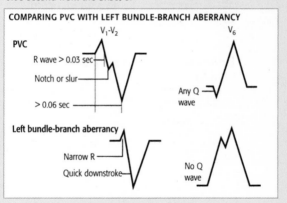

COMPARING PVC WITH LEFT BUNDLE-BRANCH ABERRANCY

NURSING INTERVENTIONS

■ Promptly assess patients with recently developed PVCs, especially if they have underlying heart disease or complex medical problems.

■ Observe closely for more frequent PVCs or more dangerous PVC patterns and notify the practitioner of changes.

■ Teach family members how to contact the emergency medical system and encourage them to learn cardiopulmonary resuscitation (CPR).

Idioventricular rhythm

Idioventricular rhythm, also referred to as ventricular escape rhythm, originates in an escape pacemaker site in the ventricles. The inherent firing rate of this ectopic pacemaker is usually 30 to 40 beats/minute. The rhythm acts as a safety mechanism by preventing ventricular standstill, or asystole—the absence of electrical activity in the ventricles. When fewer than three QRS complexes arising from the escape pacemaker occur, they're called ventricular escape beats or complexes. (See *Recognizing idioventricular rhythm.*)

RED FLAG

Recognizing idioventricular rhythm

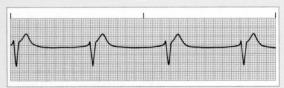

This rhythm strip illustrates idioventricular rhythm.

- *Rhythm:* regular
- *Rate:* unable to determine atrial rate; ventricular rate of 35 beats/minute
- *P wave:* absent
- *PR interval:* unmeasurable
- *QRS complex:* wide and bizarre
- *T wave:* deflection opposite QRS complex
- *QT interval:* 0.60 second
- *Other:* none

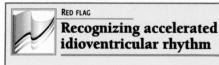

Recognizing accelerated idioventricular rhythm

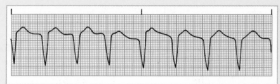

This rhythm strip illustrates accelerated idioventricular rhythm.

- *Rhythm:* regular
- *Rate:* ventricular— 80 beats/minute
- *P wave:* absent
- *PR interval:* unmeasurable
- *QRS complex:* 0.18 second; wide and bizarre
- *T wave:* directly opposite last part of QRS complex
- *QT interval:* prolonged
- *Other:* none

When the rate of an ectopic pacemaker site in the ventricles is below 100 beats/minute but exceeds the inherent ventricular escape rate of 30 to 40 beats/minute, it's called accelerated idioventricular rhythm or AIVR. (See *Recognizing accelerated idioventricular rhythm.*) The rate of AIVR isn't fast enough to be considered VT. The rhythm is usually related to enhanced automaticity of the ventricular tissue. AIVR and idioventricular rhythm share the same ECG characteristics, differing only in heart rate. Because the rate of AIVR is similar to a normal heart rate, the patient is usually asymptomatic.

CAUSES

Idioventricular rhythms occur when all of the heart's higher pacemakers fail to function or when supraventricular impulses can't reach the ventricles because of a block in the conduction system. Idioventricular rhythms may accompany third-degree heart block. Possible causes of the rhythm include:

■ myocardial ischemia

■ myocardial infarction (MI)

■ digoxin toxicity, beta blockers, calcium antagonists, and tricyclic antidepressants

■ pacemaker failure

■ metabolic imbalances.

CLINICAL SIGNIFICANCE

Idioventricular rhythm may be transient or continuous. Transient ventricular escape rhythm is usually related to increased parasympathetic effect on the higher pacemaker sites and isn't generally clinically significant. Although idioventricular rhythms act to protect the heart from ventricular standstill, a continuous idioventricular rhythm presents a clinically serious situation.

RED FLAG The slow ventricular rate of this arrhythmia and the associated loss of atrial kick markedly reduce cardiac output. If not rapidly identified and appropriately managed, idioventricular arrhythmias can cause death.

ECG CHARACTERISTICS

■ *Rhythm:* Usually, atrial rhythm can't be determined. Ventricular rhythm is usually regular.

■ *Rate:* Usually, atrial rate can't be determined. Ventricular rate is 20 to 40 beats/minute.

■ *P wave:* Absent.

■ *PR interval:* Unmeasurable because of the absent P wave.

■ *QRS complex:* Because of abnormal ventricular depolarization, the QRS complex has a duration longer than 0.12 second, with a wide and bizarre configuration.

- *T wave:* The T wave is abnormal. Deflection usually occurs in the opposite direction from that of the QRS complex.
- *QT interval:* Usually prolonged.
- *Other:* Idioventricular rhythm commonly occurs with third-degree atrioventricular block.

SIGNS AND SYMPTOMS

The patient with continuous idioventricular rhythm is generally symptomatic because of the marked reduction in cardiac output that occurs with the arrhythmia. Blood pressure may be difficult or impossible to auscultate or palpate. The patient may experience dizziness, light-headedness, syncope, or loss of consciousness.

TREATMENT

Treatment should be initiated immediately to increase the patient's heart rate, improve cardiac output, and establish a normal rhythm. Atropine may be given to increase the heart rate.

If atropine isn't effective or if the patient develops hypotension or other signs of clinical instability, a pacemaker may be needed to reestablish a heart rate that provides enough cardiac output to perfuse organs properly. A transcutaneous pacemaker may be used in an emergency until a temporary or transvenous pacemaker can be inserted. (See *Transcutaneous pacemaker,* page 148.)

RED FLAG Remember that the goal of treatment doesn't include suppressing the idioventricular rhythm because it acts as a safety mechanism to protect the heart from ventricular standstill. Idioventricular rhythm should never be treated with lidocaine or other antiarrhythmics that would suppress the escape beats.

Transcutaneous pacemaker

Transcutaneous pacing, also referred to as *external pacing* or *noninvasive pacing*, involves the delivery of electrical impulses through externally applied cutaneous electrodes. The electrical impulses are conducted through an intact chest wall using skin electrodes placed either in anterior-posterior or sternal-apex positions. (An anterior-posterior placement is shown here.)

Transcutaneous pacing is the initial pacing method of choice in emergency situations because it's the least invasive technique, and it can be instituted quickly.

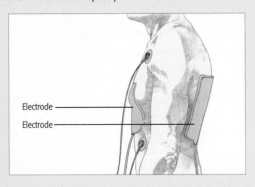

Electrode
Electrode

NURSING INTERVENTIONS
- Monitor ECG continually.
- Closely assess the patient until treatment restores hemodynamic stability.
- Keep atropine and pacemaker equipment available at the bedside.
- Enforce bed rest until an effective heart rate has been maintained and the patient is clinically stable.
- Tell the patient and his family about the serious nature of this arrhythmia and the treatment it requires.

■ If the patient needs a permanent pacemaker, teach the patient and his family how it works, how to recognize problems, when to contact the practitioner, and how pacemaker function will be monitored.

Ventricular tachycardia

VT, also called *V tach,* occurs when three or more PVCs strike in a row and the ventricular rate exceeds 100 beats/minute. This life-threatening arrhythmia usually precedes ventricular fibrillation and sudden cardiac death, especially in patients who aren't in a health care facility.

VT is an extremely unstable rhythm and may be sustained or nonsustained. When it occurs in short, paroxysmal bursts lasting under 30 seconds and causing few or no symptoms, it's called nonsustained. When the rhythm is sustained, however, it requires immediate treatment to prevent death, even in patients initially able to maintain adequate cardiac output. (See *Recognizing ventricular tachycardia,* page 150.)

CAUSES

This arrhythmia usually results from increased myocardial irritability, which may be triggered by enhanced automaticity, reentry within the Purkinje system, or by PVCs occurring during the downstroke of the preceding T wave.

Causes of VT include:

■ cardiomyopathy
■ coronary artery disease (CAD)
■ drug intoxication from procainamide, quinidine, or cocaine
■ electrolyte imbalances such as hypokalemia
■ heart failure

Recognizing ventricular tachycardia

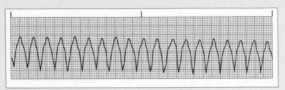

This rhythm strip illustrates ventricular tachycardia.

- *Rhythm:* regular
- *Rate:* 187 beats/minute
- *P wave:* absent
- *PR interval:* unmeasurable
- *QRS complex:* 0.16 second; wide and bizarre
- *T wave:* opposite direction of QRS complex
- *QT interval:* unmeasurable
- *Other:* none

- MI
- myocardial ischemia
- proarrhythmic effects of some antiarrhythmics
- valvular heart disease.

CLINICAL SIGNIFICANCE

VT is significant because of its unpredictability and potential for causing death. A patient may be hemodynamically stable, with a normal pulse and blood pressure; clinically unstable, with hypotension and poor peripheral pulses; or unconscious, without respirations or pulse.

Because of the reduced ventricular filling time and the drop in cardiac output that occurs with this arrhythmia, the patient's condition can quickly deteriorate to ventricular fibrillation and complete cardiovascular collapse.

ECG CHARACTERISTICS

- *Rhythm:* Atrial rhythm can't be determined. Ventricular rhythm is usually regular but may be slightly irregular.
- *Rate:* Atrial rate can't be determined. Ventricular rate is usually rapid (100 to 250 beats/minute).
- *P wave:* The P wave is usually absent. It may be obscured by the QRS complex; if identified, P waves are dissociated from the QRS complexes. Retrograde or upright P waves may be present. The presence of dissociated P waves during a wide complex tachycardia is diagnostic of VT.
- *PR interval:* Unmeasurable because the P wave can't be seen in most cases.
- *QRS complex:* Duration is greater than 0.12 second; it usually has a bizarre appearance, with increased amplitude. QRS complexes in monomorphic VT have a uniform shape. In polymorphic VT, the shape of the QRS complex constantly changes.
- *T wave:* If the T wave is visible, it occurs opposite the QRS complex.
- *QT interval:* Unmeasurable.
- *Other:* Torsades de pointes is a special variation of polymorphic VT. (See *Recognizing torsades de pointes,* page 152.)

 LIFE STAGES Torsades de pointes at an early age is usually due to congenital long-QT syndrome.

SIGNS AND SYMPTOMS

Although some patients have only minor symptoms initially, they still require rapid intervention to prevent cardiovascular collapse. Most patients with VT have weak or absent pulses. Low cardiac output will cause hypotension and a decreased level of consciousness, quickly leading to unresponsiveness if left untreated. VT may prompt angi-

Recognizing torsades de pointes

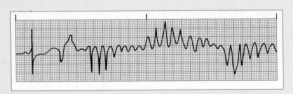

This rhythm strip illustrates torsades de pointes.

- *Rhythm:* atrial rhythm–can't be determined; ventricular rhythm–regular
- *Rate:* atrial rate–can't be determined; ventricular rate–150 to 250 beats/minute
- *P wave:* not identifiable because it's buried in the QRS complex
- *PR interval:* unmeasurable
- *QRS complex:* wide with a phasic variation in its electrical polarity
- *T wave:* not discernible
- *QT interval:* not identifiable
- *Other:* none

na, heart failure, or a substantial decrease in organ perfusion.

TREATMENT

Treatment depends on the patient's condition. Is the patient conscious? Does the patient have spontaneous respirations? Is a palpable carotid pulse present?

Patients with pulseless VT are treated the same as those with ventricular fibrillation and require immediate defibrillation and CPR. Treatment for patients with a detectable pulse depends on whether they're stable or unstable.

Unstable patients generally have ventricular rates greater than 150 beats/minute and have serious signs and symptoms related to the tachycardia, which may include:

■ hypotension
■ shortness of breath
■ chest pain
■ altered consciousness.

These patients are usually treated with immediate synchronized cardioversion.

A stable patient with VT and no signs of heart failure is treated differently. Treatment for these patients is determined by whether the rhythm is regular or irregular. If the rhythm is regular (monomorphic), the patient is treated with amiodarone and possible synchronized cardioversion. If the rate is irregular (polymorphic), look at the length of the QT interval when the rhythm is in sinus rhythm. If the QT interval is long, the polymorphic rhythm is most likely torsades de pointes. The treatment for polymorphic VT is to stop drugs that may cause a long QT, correct electrolyte imbalances, and give an antiarrhythmic, such as magnesium or amiodarone. If at any point the patient becomes unstable, immediate synchronized cardioversion is the best treatment.

Patients with VT or VF not from a transient or reversible cause may need an implanted cardioverter-defibrillator (ICD). This device is a permanent solution to recurrent episodes of VT.

A 12-lead ECG and all other available clinical information are critical for establishing a specific diagnosis in a stable patient with wide QRS complex tachycardia of unknown type but regular rate. If a definitive diagnosis of supraventricular tachycardia or VT can't be established, amiodarone (to control the rate) and elective synchronized cardioversion are used.

NURSING INTERVENTIONS

■ Determine whether the patient is conscious and has spontaneous respirations and palpable carotid pulse.
■ Initiate CPR and advanced life support measures as necessary.
■ Monitor heart rate and rhythm. The rhythm may rapidly progress to ventricular fibrillation.
■ Teach the patient and his family about the serious nature of this arrhythmia and the need for prompt treatment.
■ If your stable patient is undergoing electrical cardioversion, inform him that he'll be given a sedative, and possibly an analgesic, prior to the procedure.

RED FLAG If a patient will be discharged with an ICD or a prescription for long-term antiarrhythmics, ensure that family members know how to use the emergency medical system and how to perform CPR.

Ventricular fibrillation

Ventricular fibrillation, commonly called *V-fib* or *VF,* is characterized by a chaotic, disorganized pattern of electrical activity. The pattern arises from electrical impulses coming from multiple ectopic pacemakers in the ventricles.

The arrhythmia produces no effective ventricular mechanical activity or contractions and no cardiac output. Untreated VF is the most common cause of sudden cardiac death in people outside of a health care facility. (See *Recognizing ventricular fibrillation.*)

CAUSES

Causes include:
■ acid-base imbalance

Recognizing ventricular fibrillation

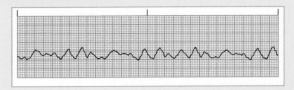

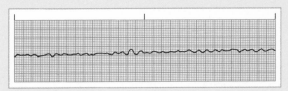

These rhythm strips illustrate ventricular fibrillation (VF).

- *Rhythm:* chaotic
- *Rate:* can't be determined
- *P wave:* absent
- *PR interval:* unmeasurable
- *QRS complex:* indiscernible
- *T wave:* indiscernible
- *QT interval:* not applicable

- *Other:* the presence of large fibrillation waves indicates coarse VF (as shown in the first electrocardiogram [ECG] strip); the presence of small fibrillation waves indicates fine VF (as shown in the second ECG strip)

- CAD
- drug toxicity, including digoxin, quinidine, and procainamide
- electric shock
- electrolyte imbalances, such as hypokalemia, hyperkalemia, and hypercalcemia
- MI
- myocardial ischemia
- severe hypothermia

- severe hypoxia
- underlying heart disease
- untreated VT.

CLINICAL SIGNIFICANCE

With VF, the ventricular muscle quivers, replacing effective muscular contraction with completely ineffective contraction. Cardiac output falls to zero and, if allowed to continue, leads to ventricular standstill and death.

ECG CHARACTERISTICS

- *Rhythm:* Atrial rhythm can't be determined. Ventricular rhythm has no pattern or regularity. Ventricular electrical activity appears as fibrillatory waves with no recognizable pattern.
- *Rate:* Atrial and ventricular rates can't be determined.
- *P wave:* Can't be determined.
- *PR interval:* Can't be determined.
- *QRS complex:* Duration can't be determined.
- *T wave:* Can't be determined.
- *QT interval:* Not applicable.
- *Other:* Coarse fibrillation waves are generally associated with greater chances of successful electrical cardioversion than smaller amplitude waves. Fibrillation waves become finer as hypoxemia and acidosis progress, making the VF more resistant to defibrillation.

SIGNS AND SYMPTOMS

The patient in VF is in full cardiac arrest, unresponsive, and without a detectable blood pressure or central pulses. Whenever you see an ECG pattern resembling VF, check the patient immediately and initiate definitive treatment.

TREATMENT

Immediate defibrillation and CPR are the most effective treatments for VF. CPR must be performed until the defibrillator arrives (to preserve oxygen supply to the brain and other vital organs) and after the first attempt at defibrillation. After a cycle of CPR, a second defibrillation is attempted. Defibrillators vary by facility and may deliver monophasic or biphasic current. (See *Monophasic and biphasic defibrillators*, page 158.)

Drugs, such as epinephrine and vasopressin, may be used for persistent VF if the first two attempts at defibrillation are unsuccessful. Antiarrhythmics, such as amiodarone, lidocaine, and magnesium, may also be considered. (For specific treatment, see the ACLS pulseless arrest algorithm, pages 262 and 263.) In defibrillation, two electrode paddles or pads are applied to the chest wall. Current is then directed through the pads and, subsequently, the patient's chest and heart. The current causes the myocardium to completely depolarize, which, in turn, encourages the SA node to resume normal control of the heart's electrical activity.

For anterolateral placement, one electrode paddle or pad is placed to the right of the upper sternum, and one is placed over the fifth or sixth intercostal space at the left anterior axillary line. For anteroposterior placement, one electrode paddle or pad is placed directly over the heart at the precordium, to the left of the sternal border, and one is placed under the patient's body beneath the heart and just below the left scapula. During cardiac surgery, internal paddles are placed directly on the myocardium.

Automated external defibrillators (AEDs) are increasingly being used, especially outside of the hospital, to provide early defibrillation. After a patient is confirmed to be unresponsive, breathless, and pulseless, the AED power is turned on and the electrode pads and cables at-

Monophasic and biphasic defibrillators

MONOPHASIC DEFIBRILLATORS

Monophasic defibrillators deliver a single current of electricity that travels  in one direction between the two pads or paddles on the patient's chest. To be effective, a large amount of electrical current is required for monophasic defibrillation.

BIPHASIC DEFIBRILLATORS

Biphasic defibrillators have the same pad or paddle placement as with the monophasic defibrillator. The difference is that during biphasic defibrillation, the electrical current discharged from the pads or paddles travels in a positive direction for a specified duration and then reverses and flows in a negative direction for the remaining time of the electrical discharge.

ENERGY EFFICIENT

The biphasic defibrillator delivers two currents of electricity and lowers the defibrillation threshold of the heart muscle, making it possible to successfully defibrillate ventricular fibrillation (VF) with smaller amounts of energy.

ADJUSTABLE

The biphasic defibrillator can adjust for differences in impedance or resistance of the current through the chest. This reduces the number of shocks needed to terminate VF.

LESS MYOCARDIAL DAMAGE

Because the biphasic defibrillator requires lower energy levels and fewer shocks, damage to the myocardial muscle is reduced. Biphasic defibrillators used at the clinically appropriate energy level may be used for defibrillation and, in the synchronized mode, for synchronized cardioversion.

tached. The AED can analyze the patient's cardiac rhythm and provide the caregiver with step-by-step instructions on how to proceed. These defibrillators can be used by people without medical experience as long as they're

Automated external defibrillator

Automated external defibrillators (AEDs) vary with the manufacturer, but the basic components of each device are similar. This illustration shows a typical AED and how to place electrodes properly.

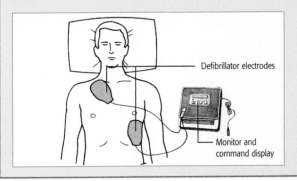

Defibrillator electrodes

Monitor and command display

trained in the proper use of the device. (See *Automated external defibrillator.*)

NURSING INTERVENTIONS

■ When faced with a rhythm that appears to be VF, always assess the patient first. Other events can mimic VF on an ECG strip, including interference from an electric razor, shivering, or seizure activity.

■ Start CPR.

■ Teach the patient and his family how to use the emergency medical system following discharge from the facility. Family members may need instruction in CPR.

■ Teach the patient and his family about long-term therapies that help prevent recurrent episodes of VF, including antiarrhythmics and ICDs.

Asystole

Ventricular asystole, also called *asystole* and *ventricular standstill,* is the absence of discernable electrical activity in the ventricles. Although some electrical activity may be evident in the atria, these impulses aren't conducted to the ventricles. (See *Recognizing asystole.*)

Asystole usually results from a prolonged period of cardiac arrest without effective resuscitation.

> **RED FLAG** *It's important to distinguish asystole from fine VF, which is managed differently. Therefore, asystole must be confirmed in more than one ECG lead.*

CAUSES
Possible, reversible causes include:
- drug overdose
- cardiac tamponade
- hypothermia
- hypovolemia
- hypoxia
- massive pulmonary embolism
- MI (coronary thrombosis)
- severe electrolyte disturbances, especially hyperkalemia and hypokalemia
- severe, uncorrected acid-base disturbances, especially metabolic acidosis
- tension pneumothorax.

CLINICAL SIGNIFICANCE
Without ventricular electrical activity, ventricular contractions can't occur. As a result, cardiac output drops to zero and vital organs are no longer perfused. Asystole has been called the arrhythmia of death and is typically considered to be a confirmation of death, rather than an arrhythmia to be treated.

Recognizing asystole

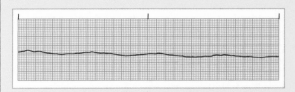

This rhythm strip illustrates asystole.

- *Rhythm:* atrial rhythm—indiscernible; no ventricular rhythm
- *Rate:* atrial rate—indiscernible; no ventricular rate
- *P wave:* not present
- *PR interval:* unmeasurable
- *QRS complex:* absent
- *T wave:* absent
- *QT interval:* unmeasurable
- *Other:* absence of electrical activity in the ventricles results in a nearly flat line

The patient with asystole is completely unresponsive, without spontaneous respirations or pulse (cardiopulmonary arrest). Without immediate start of CPR and rapid identification and treatment of the underlying cause, the condition quickly becomes irreversible.

ECG CHARACTERISTICS

- *Rhythm:* Atrial rhythm is usually indiscernible; no ventricular rhythm is present.
- *Rate:* Atrial rate is usually indiscernible; no ventricular rate is present.
- *P wave:* May be present.
- *PR interval:* Unmeasurable.
- *QRS complex:* Absent or occasional escape beats.
- *T wave:* Absent.
- *QT interval:* Unmeasurable.

Pulseless electrical activity

Pulseless electrical activity (PEA) defines a group of arrhythmias characterized by the presence of some type of electrical activity but no detectable pulse. Although organized electrical depolarization occurs, no synchronous shortening of the myocardial fibers occurs. As a result, no mechanical activity or contractions take place. Included in the PEA category are electromechanical dissociation (EMD), pseudo-EMD, idioventricular rhythms, and ventricular escape rhythms.

massive pulmonary embolism, hypothermia, hyperkalemia and hypokalemia, massive acute myocardial infarction, and overdoses of drugs such as tricyclic antidepressants.

TREATMENT
Rapid identification and treatment of underlying reversible causes is critical for treating PEA. For example, hypovolemia is treated with volume expansion. Tension pneumothorax is treated with needle decompression.

Institute cardiopulmonary resuscitation immediately and administer I.V. or intraosseous epinephrine or vasopressin. Atropine may be given if the PEA rate is slow.

CAUSES
The most common causes of PEA include hypovolemia, hypoxia, acidosis, tension pneumothorax, cardiac tamponade,

■ *Other:* On a rhythm strip, asystole looks like a nearly flat line (except for changes caused by chest compressions during CPR). In a patient with a pacemaker, pacer spikes may be evident on the strip but no P wave or QRS complex occurs in response to the stimulus.

SIGNS AND SYMPTOMS

The patient will be unresponsive and have no spontaneous respirations, discernible pulse, or blood pressure.

TREATMENT

Immediate treatment includes effective CPR and supplemental oxygen. Resuscitation should be attempted unless evidence exists that these efforts shouldn't be initiated such as when a do-not-resuscitate (DNR) order is in effect. (See the ACLS pulseless arrest algorithm, pages 262 and 263.)

Priority must also be given to searching for and treating identified potentially reversible causes. Early CPR is vital, and I.V. or intraosseous epinephrine or a one-time dose of vasopressin and atropine is given.

Pulseless electrical activity can also lead to asystole. (See *Pulseless electrical activity*.)

With persistent asystole despite appropriate intervention, consideration should be given to stopping resuscitation.

NURSING INTERVENTIONS

- Verify the presence of asystole by checking more than one ECG lead.
- Verify lack of DNR order.
- Start CPR and advanced life support measures.

7

ATRIOVENTRICULAR BLOCKS

Atrioventricular (AV) heart block refers to a permanent or transient interruption or delay in the conduction of electrical impulses between the atria and the ventricles. The block can occur at the AV node, the bundle of His, or the bundle branches. When the site of the block is the bundle of His or the bundle branches, the block is called an infranodal AV block. AV block can be partial (first or second degree) or complete (third degree).

The heart's electrical impulses normally originate in the sinoatrial (SA) node, so when those impulses are blocked at the AV node, atrial rates are typically normal (60 to 100 beats/minute). The significance of the block depends on the number of impulses completely blocked and the resulting ventricular rate. A slow ventricular rate can decrease cardiac output and cause such symptoms as light-headedness, hypotension, and altered mental status.

CAUSES OF AV BLOCK

A variety of factors may lead to AV block, including underlying heart conditions, use of certain drugs, congenital anomalies, and conditions that disrupt the cardiac conduction system.

Typical causes of AV block include:
- myocardial ischemia, which impairs cellular function so that cells repolarize more slowly or incompletely.

The injured cells, in turn, may conduct impulses slowly or inconsistently. Relief of the ischemia may restore normal function to the AV node.

■ myocardial infarction (MI), in which cellular necrosis or death occurs. If the necrotic cells are part of the conduction system, they may no longer conduct impulses and a permanent AV block occurs.

■ excessive levels of, or an exaggerated response to, a drug. This response can cause AV block or increase the likelihood that a block will develop. The drugs may increase the refractory period of a portion of the conduction system. Although many antiarrhythmics can have this effect, the drugs more commonly known to cause or exacerbate AV blocks include digoxin, beta and calcium channel blockers, and amiodarone.

■ lesions, including calcium and fibrotic lesions, along the conduction pathway.

■ congenital anomalies such as congenital ventricular septal defects that involve cardiac structures and affect the conduction system. Anomalies of the conduction system, such as an AV node that doesn't conduct impulses, can also occur in the absence of structural defects.

■ increased vagal tone due to pain, carotid sinus massage, or a hypersensitive carotid sinus can slow the sinus node and lead to an AV block.

■ cardiomyopathies, myocarditis, and cardiac tumors.

LIFE STAGES *In elderly patients, AV block may be due to fibrosis of the conduction system. Other causes include the use of digoxin and the presence of aortic valve calcification.*

AV block can also be caused by inadvertent damage to the heart's conduction system during cardiac surgery. Damage is most likely to occur in operations involving the mitral or tricuspid valve or in the closure of a ventricular septal defect. If the injury involves tissues adjacent to the surgical site and the conduction system isn't physically disrupted, the block may be only temporary. If a portion of the conduction system itself is severed, permanent block results.

Similar disruption of the conduction system can occur from a procedure called radiofrequency ablation. In this invasive procedure, a transvenous catheter is used to locate the area in the heart that participates in initiating or perpetuating certain tachyarrhythmias. Radiofrequency energy is then delivered to the myocardium through this catheter to produce a small area of necrosis at that spot. The damaged tissue can no longer cause or participate in the tachyarrhythmia. If the energy is delivered close to the AV node, bundle of His, or bundle branches, AV block can result.

CLASSIFYING AV BLOCK

AV blocks are classified by the site of block and the severity of the conduction abnormality. The sites of AV block include the AV node, bundle of His, and bundle branches.

Severity of AV block is classified in degrees:
■ first-degree AV block
■ second-degree AV block
  – type I (Wenckebach or Mobitz I, after the scientists who first identified them)
  – type II (Mobitz II) AV block
■ third-degree (complete) AV block.

The classification system for AV blocks aids in the determination of the patient's treatment and prognosis.

First-degree AV block

First-degree AV block occurs when there's a delay in the conduction of electrical impulses from the atria to the ventricles. This delay usually occurs at the level of the AV node, but it may also be infranodal. First-degree AV block is characterized by a PR interval greater than 0.20 second. This interval usually remains constant beat to beat. Electrical impulses are conducted through the normal conduction pathway. However, conduction of these impulses takes longer than normal.

CAUSES

First-degree AV block may result from:
■ myocardial ischemia or MI
■ myocarditis
■ degenerative changes in the heart associated with aging.
  The condition may also be caused by drugs, such as:
■ digoxin
■ calcium channel blockers
■ beta blockers.

CLINICAL SIGNIFICANCE

A healthy person with first-degree AV block may be asymptomatic. The arrhythmia may be transient, especially if it occurs secondary to drugs or ischemia early in the course of an MI. The presence of first-degree block, the least dangerous type of AV block, indicates a delay in the conduction of electrical impulses through the normal conduction pathway. In general, a rhythm strip with this block looks like normal sinus rhythm except that the PR interval is longer than normal.

RED FLAG Because first-degree AV block can progress to a more severe type of AV block, the patient's cardiac rhythm should be monitored for changes. (See *Recognizing first-degree atrioventricular block,* page 168.)

ECG CHARACTERISTICS

■ *Rhythm:* Atrial and ventricular rhythms are regular.

Recognizing first-degree atrioventricular block

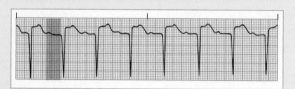

This rhythm strip illustrates first-degree atrioventricular block.

- *Rhythm:* regular
- *Rate:* 75 beats/minute
- *P wave:* normal
- *PR interval:* 0.32 second; greater than 0.20 second (see shaded area)
- *QRS complex:* 0.08 second
- *T wave:* normal
- *QT interval:* 0.40 second
- *Other:* PR interval—prolonged but constant

■ *Rate:* Atrial and ventricular rates are the same and within normal limits.

■ *P wave:* Normal size and configuration; each P wave followed by a QRS complex.

■ *PR interval:* Prolonged (greater than 0.20 second) but constant.

■ *QRS complex:* Duration usually remains within normal limits if the conduction delay occurs in the AV node. If the QRS duration exceeds 0.12 second, the conduction delay may be in the His-Purkinje system.

■ *T wave:* Normal size and configuration unless the QRS complex is prolonged.

■ *QT interval:* Usually within normal limits.

■ *Other:* None.

SIGNS AND SYMPTOMS

The patient's pulse rate will usually be normal, and the rhythm will be regular. Most patients with first-degree AV block are asymptomatic because cardiac output isn't significantly affected. If the PR interval is extremely long, a longer interval between S_1 and S_2 may be noticed during auscultation.

TREATMENT

Treatment generally focuses on identification and correction of the underlying cause. For example, if a drug is causing the AV block, the dosage may be reduced or the drug stopped. Close monitoring can help detect progressive prolongation of the PR interval or progression of first-degree AV block to a more serious form of block.

NURSING INTERVENTIONS

- Observe the electrocardiogram (ECG) for progression of the block to a more severe form.
- Administer digoxin, calcium channel blockers, and beta blockers cautiously.

Type I second-degree AV block

Also called *Wenckebach* or *Mobitz I block,* type I second-degree AV block occurs when each successive impulse from the SA node is delayed slightly longer than the previous impulse. (See *Recognizing type I second-degree atrioventricular block,* page 170.) This pattern of progressive prolongation of the PR interval continues until an impulse fails to be conducted to the ventricles.

Usually only a single impulse is blocked from reaching the ventricles, and following this nonconducted

Recognizing type I second-degree atrioventricular block

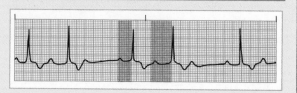

This rhythm strip illustrates type I second-degree atrioventricular block.

- *Rhythm:* atrial—regular; ventricular—irregular
- *Rate:* atrial—80 beats/minute; ventricular—50 beats/minute
- *P wave:* normal
- *PR interval:* progressively prolonged (see shaded areas)
- *QRS complex:* 0.08 second
- *T wave:* inverted
- *QT interval:* 0.46 second
- *Other:* Wenckebach pattern of grouped beats; the PR interval gets progressively longer until a QRS complex is dropped

P wave or dropped beat, the pattern is repeated. This repetitive sequence of two or more consecutive beats followed by a dropped beat results in "group beating." Type I second-degree AV block generally occurs at the level of the AV node.

CAUSES

Type I second-degree AV block frequently results from increased parasympathetic tone or the effects of certain drugs. Coronary artery disease (CAD), inferior-wall MI, and rheumatic fever may increase parasympathetic tone and result in the arrhythmia. It may also be due to cardiac drugs, such as beta blockers, digoxin, and calcium channel blockers.

CLINICAL SIGNIFICANCE

Type I second-degree AV block may occur normally in an otherwise healthy person. It may also occur in patients with a high vagal tone, in athletes at rest, or in elderly patients. Almost always transient, this type of block usually resolves when the underlying condition is corrected. Although an asymptomatic patient with this block has a good prognosis, the block may progress to a more serious form, especially if it occurs early in an MI.

ECG CHARACTERISTICS

■ *Rhythm:* Atrial rhythm is regular, and the ventricular rhythm is irregular. The R-R interval shortens progressively until a P wave appears without a QRS complex. The cycle is then repeated.

■ *Rate:* The atrial rate exceeds the ventricular rate because of the nonconducted beats, but both usually remain within normal limits.

■ *P wave:* Normal size and configuration; each P wave is followed by a QRS complex except for the blocked P wave.

■ *PR interval:* The PR interval is progressively longer with each cycle until a P wave appears without a QRS complex. The variation in delay from cycle to cycle is typically slight. The PR interval after the nonconducted beat is shorter than the interval preceding it. The phrase commonly used to describe this pattern is long, longer, dropped.

■ *QRS complex:* Duration usually remains within normal limits because the block commonly occurs at the level of the AV node. The complex is periodically absent.

■ *T wave:* Normal size and configuration, but its deflection may be opposite that of the QRS complex.

■ *QT interval:* Usually within normal limits.

■ *Other:* The arrhythmia is usually distinguished by group beating, referred to as the *footprints of Wencke-bach.*

SIGNS AND SYMPTOMS

Usually asymptomatic, a patient with type I second-degree AV block may show signs and symptoms of decreased cardiac output, such as light-headedness or hypotension. Symptoms may be especially pronounced if the ventricular rate is slow.

TREATMENT

Treatment is rarely needed because the patient is generally asymptomatic. For a patient with serious signs and symptoms related to a low heart rate, atropine may be used to improve AV node conduction. A transcutaneous pacemaker may be required for a symptomatic patient until the arrhythmia resolves. (See Bradycardia algorithm, pages 260 and 261.)

NURSING INTERVENTIONS

■ Check the ECG frequently to see if a more severe type of AV block develops.
■ Monitor the tolerance for the rhythm.
■ Observe for signs and symptoms of decreased cardiac output.
■ Provide patient teaching about a temporary pacemaker if indicated.

Type II second-degree AV block

Type II second-degree AV block (also known as Mobitz II block) is less common than type I, but more serious. It occurs when impulses from the SA node occasionally fail

RED FLAG

Recognizing type II second-degree atrioventricular block

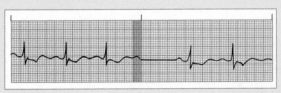

This rhythm illustrates type II second-degree atrioventricular block.

- *Rhythm:* atrial—regular; ventricular—irregular
- *Rate:* atrial—60 beats/minute; ventricular—50 beats/minute
- *P wave:* normal
- *PR interval:* 0.28 second; the PR interval is constant for the conducted beats

- *QRS complex:* 0.10 second
- *T wave:* normal
- *QT interval:* 0.60 second
- *Other:* PR and R-R intervals don't vary before a dropped beat (see shaded area), so no warning occurs

to conduct to the ventricles. This form of second-degree AV block occurs below the level of the AV node, either at the bundle of His, or more commonly at the bundle branches.

One of the hallmarks of this type of block is that, unlike type I second-degree AV block, the PR interval doesn't lengthen before a dropped beat. (See *Recognizing type II second-degree atrioventricular block*.) In addition, more than one nonconducted beat can occur in succession.

CAUSES

Unlike type I second-degree AV block, type II second-degree AV block rarely results from increased parasympathetic tone or drug effect. Because the arrhythmia is usually associated with organic heart disease and, therefore, a poorer prognosis—complete heart block may develop.

Type II second-degree AV block is commonly caused by:

■ an anterior-wall MI
■ degenerative changes in the conduction system
■ severe CAD.

CLINICAL SIGNIFICANCE

Unlike type I second-degree AV block, type II second-degree AV block rarely results from increased parasympathetic tone or drug effect, and it almost always occurs below the AV node. As a result, this type of block is usually associated with a poorer prognosis and a greater probability that complete heart block may develop.

In type II second-degree AV block, the ventricular rate tends to be slower than in type I. In addition, cardiac output tends to be lower and symptoms are more likely to appear, particularly if the sinus rhythm is slow and the ratio of conducted beats to dropped beats is low such as 2:1.

ECG CHARACTERISTICS

■ *Rhythm:* The atrial rhythm is regular. The ventricular rhythm can be regular or irregular. Pauses correspond to the dropped beat. When the block is intermittent or when the conduction ratio is variable, the rhythm is commonly irregular. When a constant conduction ratio occurs, for example, 2:1 or 3:1, the rhythm is regular.
■ *Rate:* The atrial rate is usually within normal limits. The ventricular rate, slower than the atrial rate, may be within normal limits.
■ *P wave:* The P wave is normal in size and configuration, but some P waves aren't followed by a QRS complex.

The R-R interval containing a nonconducted P wave equals two normal R-R intervals.

■ *PR interval:* The PR interval is within normal limits or prolonged but generally always constant for the conducted beats. It may be shortened if following a nonconducted beat.

■ *QRS complex:* Duration is within normal limits if the block occurs at the bundle of His. If the block occurs at the bundle branches, however, the QRS will be widened and display the features of bundle-branch block. The complex is absent periodically.

■ *T wave:* Usually of normal size and configuration.

■ *QT interval:* Usually within normal limits.

■ *Other:* The PR and R-R intervals don't vary before a dropped beat, so no warning occurs. The R-R interval that contains the nonconducted P wave equals two normal R-R intervals. For a dropped beat to occur, there must be complete block in one bundle branch with intermittent interruption in conduction in the other bundle as well.

SIGNS AND SYMPTOMS

Most patients who experience occasional dropped beats remain asymptomatic as long as cardiac output is maintained. As the number of dropped beats increases, the patient may experience signs and symptoms of decreased cardiac output, including:

■ fatigue
■ dyspnea
■ chest pain
■ light-headedness
■ syncope
■ altered mental status.

On assessment, you may note hypotension and a slow pulse, with a regular or irregular rhythm.

TREATMENTS

If the patient doesn't experience serious signs and symptoms related to the low heart rate, the patient may be prepared for transvenous pacemaker insertion. Or the patient may be continuously monitored with a transcutaneous pacemaker.

If the patient is experiencing serious signs and symptoms due to bradycardia, treatment goals include improving cardiac output by increasing the heart rate. I.V. atropine, transcutaneous pacing, I.V. dopamine, or I.V. epinephrine may be used to increase cardiac output. (See Bradycardia algorithm, pages 260 and 261.)

Because this form of second-degree AV block occurs below the level of the AV node— either at the bundle of His or, more commonly, at the bundle branches—transcutaneous pacing should be initiated quickly, when indicated. For this reason, type II second-degree AV block may also require placement of a permanent pacemaker. A temporary pacemaker may be used until a permanent pacemaker can be inserted.

NURSING INTERVENTIONS

- Observe cardiac rhythm for progression to a more severe form of AV block.
- Assess tolerance for the rhythm and the need for treatment to improve cardiac output.
- Keep the patient on bed rest, if indicated, to reduce myocardial oxygen demands.
- Give oxygen therapy as indicated.
- Keep transcutaneous pacemaker at the bedside as indicated.
- Teach the patient and his family about the use of pacemakers if the patient requires one.

Third-degree AV block

Also called complete heart block or AV dissociation, third-degree AV block indicates the complete absence of impulse conduction between the atria and ventricles. In complete heart block, the atrial rate is generally equal to or faster than the ventricular rate.

Third-degree AV block may occur at the level of the AV node, the bundle of His, or the bundle branches. The patient's treatment and prognosis vary depending on the anatomic level of the block.

When third-degree AV block occurs at the level of the AV node, ventricular depolarization is typically initiated by a junctional escape pacemaker. This pacemaker is usually stable with a rate of 40 to 60 beats/minute. (See *Recognizing third-degree atrioventricular block,* page 178.) The sequence of ventricular depolarization is usually normal because the block is located above the bifurcation of the bundle of His, which results in a normal-appearing QRS complex.

On the other hand, when third-degree AV block occurs at the infranodal level, a block involving the right and left bundle branches is most commonly the cause. In this case, extensive disease exists in the infranodal conduction system, and the only available escape mechanism is located distal to the site of block in the ventricle. This unstable, ventricular escape pacemaker has a slow intrinsic rate of less than 40 beats/minute. Because these depolarizations originate in the ventricle, the QRS complex will have a wide and bizarre appearance.

CAUSES

Third-degree AV block occurring at the anatomic level of the AV node can result from:

Recognizing third-degree atrioventricular block

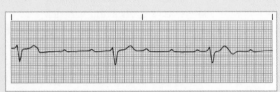

This rhythm strip illustrates third-degree atrioventricular block:

- *Rhythm:* regular
- *Rate:* atrial—90 beats/minute; ventricular—30 beats/minute
- *P wave:* normal
- *PR interval:* varied
- *QRS complex:* 0.16 second
- *T wave:* normal
- *QT interval:* 0.56 second
- *Other:* P waves occur without a QRS complex

- increased parasympathetic tone associated with inferior wall MI
- AV node damage
- toxic effects of drugs, such as digoxin and propranolol.

Third-degree AV block occurring at the infranodal level is frequently associated with extensive anterior MI. It generally isn't the result of increases in parasympathetic tone or drug effect.

LIFE STAGES *After repair of a ventricular septal defect, a child may require a permanent pacemaker if complete heart block develops. This arrhythmia may develop from interference with the bundle of His during surgery.*

CLINICAL SIGNIFICANCE

Third-degree AV block occurring at the AV node, with a junctional escape rhythm, is usually transient and generally associated with a favorable prognosis. In third-degree

AV block at the infranodal level, however, the pacemaker is unstable and episodes of ventricular asystole are common. Third-degree AV block at this level is generally associated with a less favorable prognosis.

Because the ventricular rate in third-degree AV block can be slow and the decrease in cardiac output so significant, the arrhythmia usually results in a life-threatening situation. In addition, the loss of AV synchrony results in the loss of atrial kick, which further decreases cardiac output.

ECG CHARACTERISTICS

■ *Rhythm:* Atrial and ventricular rhythms are usually regular.

■ *Rate:* Acting independently, the atria, generally under the control of the SA node, tend to maintain a regular rate of 60 to 100 beats/minute. The atrial rate exceeds the ventricular rate. With intranodal block, the ventricular rate is usually 40 to 60 beats/minute (a junctional escape rhythm). With infranodal block, the ventricular rate is usually below 40 beats/minute (a ventricular escape rhythm).

■ *P wave:* The P wave is normal in size and configuration. Some P waves may be buried in QRS complexes or T waves.

■ *PR interval:* Not applicable or measurable because the atria and ventricles are depolarized from different pacemakers and beat independently of each other (AV dissociation).

■ *QRS complex:* Configuration depends on the location of the escape mechanism and origin of ventricular depolarization. When the block occurs at the level of the AV node or bundle of His, the QRS complex will appear normal. When the block occurs at the level of the bundle branches, the QRS will be widened.

- *T wave:* Normal size and configuration unless the QRS complex originates in the ventricle.
- *QT interval:* May be within normal limits.
- *Other:* None.

SIGNS AND SYMPTOMS

Most patients with third-degree AV block experience significant signs and symptoms, including:

- severe fatigue
- dyspnea
- chest pain
- light-headedness
- changes in mental status
- changes in the level of consciousness.

Hypotension, pallor, and diaphoresis may also occur. The peripheral pulse rate will be slow, but the rhythm will be regular.

A few patients will be relatively free of symptoms, complaining only that they can't tolerate exercise and that they're typically tired for no apparent reason. The severity of symptoms depends to a large extent on the resulting ventricular rate and the patient's ability to compensate for decreased cardiac output.

TREATMENT

If the patient has serious signs and symptoms related to the low heart rate, or if the patient's condition seems to be deteriorating, interventions may include transcutaneous pacing or I.V. dopamine or epinephrine.

Asymptomatic patients with third-degree AV block should be prepared for insertion of a transvenous temporary pacemaker until a decision is made about the need for a permanent pacemaker. If symptoms develop, a transcutaneous pacemaker should be used until the transvenous pacemaker is placed.

Because third-degree AV block occurring at the infra-nodal level is usually associated with extensive anterior MI, patients are more likely to have permanent third-degree AV block, which most likely requires insertion of a permanent pacemaker.

Third-degree AV block occurring at the anatomic level of the AV node can result from increased parasympathetic tone associated with an inferior wall MI. As a result, the block is more likely to be short-lived. In these patients, the decision to insert a permanent pacemaker is usually delayed to assess how well the conduction system recovers.

NURSING INTERVENTIONS
■ Assess the patient's tolerance of the rhythm and the need for interventions to support cardiac output and relieve symptoms.
■ Make sure that the patient's I.V. line is patent.
■ Administer oxygen therapy as indicated.
■ Minimize the patient's activity and maintain bed rest.

8

PHARMACOLOGIC TREATMENTS

Almost half a million Americans die each year from arrhythmias; countless others experience symptoms and lifestyle changes. Along with other treatments, drugs can help:

- alleviate symptoms
- control heart rate and rhythm
- decrease preload and afterload
- prolong life.

Antiarrhythmics affect the movement of ions across the cell membrane and alter the electrophysiology of the cardiac cell. These drugs are classified by their effect on the cell's electrical activity (action potential) and their mechanism of action. Because the drugs can cause changes in the myocardial action potential, characteristic electrocardiogram (ECG) changes can occur. (See *Antiarrhythmics and the action potential*.)

The classification system divides antiarrhythmics into four major classes based on their dominant mechanism of action: class I, class II, class III, and class IV. Class I antiarrhythmics are further divided into class IA, class IB, and class IC.

Certain antiarrhythmics can't be classified specifically into one group. For example, sotalol possesses characteristics of both class II and class III drugs. Still, other drugs,

Antiarrhythmics and the action potential

Each class of antiarrhythmics acts on a different phase of the action potential and alters the heart's electrophysiology. Below is a summary of the four classes of antiarrhythmics and how each class affects the action potential.

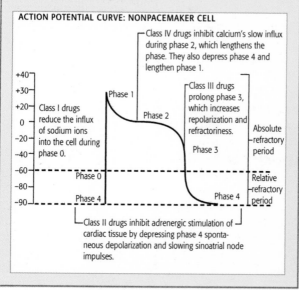

ACTION POTENTIAL CURVE: NONPACEMAKER CELL

Class IV drugs inhibit calcium's slow influx during phase 2, which lengthens the phase. They also depress phase 4 and lengthen phase 1.

Class III drugs prolong phase 3, which increases repolarization and refractoriness.

Class I drugs reduce the influx of sodium ions into the cell during phase 0.

Phase 1

Phase 2

Phase 3

Phase 0

Phase 4

Absolute refractory period

Relative refractory period

Class II drugs inhibit adrenergic stimulation of cardiac tissue by depressing phase 4 spontaneous depolarization and slowing sinoatrial node impulses.

such as adenosine, digoxin, atropine, epinephrine, and magnesium, don't fit into the classification system at all. Despite its limitations, the classification system is helpful in understanding how antiarrhythmics prevent and treat arrhythmias.

This chapter reviews ECG changes in patients taking therapeutic doses of antiarrhythmics (separated by classification) and digoxin. When levels are toxic, ECG changes are typically exaggerated.

Class I antiarrhythmics

Class I drugs block the influx of sodium into the cell during phase 0 of the action potential. Because phase 0 is also referred to as the sodium channel or fast channel, these drugs may also be called *sodium channel blockers* or *fast channel blockers*. Class I drugs are frequently subdivided into three groups—A, B, and C—according to their interactions with cardiac sodium channels or the drug's effects on the duration of the action potential.

CLASS IA
Class IA drugs include disopyramide, procainamide, and quinidine. These drugs lengthen the duration of the action potential, and their interaction with the sodium channels is classified as intermediate. As a result, conductivity is reduced and repolarization is prolonged. With the introduction of many new drugs, class IA antiarrhythmics aren't used as frequently.

ECG characteristics
■ *QRS complex:* Slightly widened; increased widening is an early sign of toxicity.
■ *T wave:* May be flattened or inverted.
■ *U wave:* May be present.
■ *QT interval:* Prolonged.
    Because these drugs prolong the QT interval, the patient is prone to polymorphic ventricular tachycardia. (See *ECG effects of class IA antiarrhythmics.*)

CLASS IB
Class IB agents include phenytoin, lidocaine, and mexiletine. These drugs interact rapidly with sodium channels, slowing phase 0 of the action potential and shortening

ECG effects of class IA antiarrhythmics

Class IA antiarrhythmics—including quinidine and procainamide—affect the cardiac cycle in specific ways and lead to specific electrocardiogram (ECG) changes, as shown below. Class IA antiarrhythmics:

- block sodium influx during phase 0, depressing the rate of depolarization
- prolong repolarization and the duration of the action potential
- lengthen the refractory period
- decrease contractility.

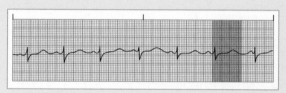

ECG characteristics (see shaded area) of class IA antiarrhythmics:

- *QRS complex:* slightly widened
- *QT interval:* prolonged

phase 3. The drugs in this class are effective in suppressing ventricular ectopy.

ECG characteristics

- *PR interval:* May be slightly shortened.
- *QT interval:* Shortened. (See *ECG effects of class IB antiarrhythmics,* page 186.)

CLASS IC

Class IC drugs include flecainide and propafenone and may minimally increase or have no effect on the action potential duration. They interact slowly with sodium

ECG effects of class IB antiarrhythmics

Class IB antiarrhythmics—such as lidocaine and tocainide—may affect the QRS complex, as shown on the rhythm strip below. The drugs may also:
- block sodium influx during phase 0, depressing the rate of depolarization
- shorten repolarization and the duration of the action potential
- suppress ventricular automaticity in ischemic tissue.

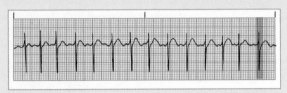

Electrocardiogram (ECG) characteristics of class IB antiarrhythmics:
- *PR interval:* prolonged
- *QRS complex:* slightly widened (see shaded area)

channels. Phase 0 is markedly slowed and conduction is decreased.

These antiarrhythmics are generally reserved for refractory arrhythmias because they may cause or worsen arrhythmias. (See *ECG effects of class IC antiarrhythmics.*)

ECG characteristics
- ▪ *PR interval:* Prolonged.
- ▪ *QRS complex:* Widened.
- ▪ *QT interval:* Prolonged.

ECG effects of class IC antiarrhythmics

Class IC antiarrhythmics—including flecainide and propafenone—cause the effects shown below on an electrocardiogram (ECG) by exerting particular actions on the cardiac cycle. Class IC antiarrhythmics block sodium influx during phase 0, which depresses the rate of depolarization. The drugs exert no effect on repolarization or the duration of the action potential.

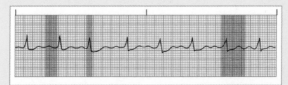

ECG characteristics of class IC antiarrhythmics:
- *PR interval:* prolonged (see shaded area above left)
- *QRS complex:* widened (see shaded area above center)
- *QT interval:* prolonged (see shaded area above right)

Class II antiarrhythmics

Class II antiarrhythmics include drugs that reduce adrenergic activity in the heart. Beta antagonists, also called *beta-adrenergic blockers*, are class II antiarrhythmics and include such drugs as metoprolol and propranolol. Beta blockers block beta receptors in the sympathetic nervous system. As a result, phase 4 depolarization is diminished, which leads to depressed automaticity of the sinoatrial (SA) node and increased atrial and atrioventricular (AV) node refractory periods.

Class II drugs are used to treat supraventricular and ventricular arrhythmias, especially those caused by excess

ECG effects of class II antiarrhythmics

Class II antiarrhythmics—including beta blockers, such as propranolol and esmolol—cause certain effects on an electrocardiogram (ECG) (as shown here) by exerting particular actions on the cardiac cycle. Class II antiarrhythmics:

- depress sinoatrial node automaticity
- shorten the duration of the action potential
- increase the refractory period of atrial and atrioventricular junctional tissues, which slows conduction
- inhibit sympathetic activity.

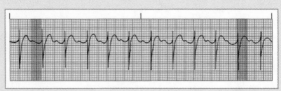

ECG characteristics of class II antiarrhythmics:

- *PR interval:* slightly prolonged (see shaded area above left)
- *QT interval:* slightly shortened (see shaded area above right)

circulating catecholamines. Beta blockers are classified according to their effects. Beta$_1$ blockers decrease:

- heart rate
- contractility
- conductivity.

Beta$_2$ blockers may cause vasoconstriction and bronchospasm because beta$_2$ receptors relax smooth muscle in the bronchi and blood vessels.

Beta-adrenergic blockers that block only beta$_1$ receptors are referred to as cardioselective. Those that have both beta$_1$- and beta$_2$-receptor activity are referred to as noncardioselective.

ECG CHARACTERISTICS

- ■ *Rate:* Atrial and ventricular rates are decreased.
- ■ *PR interval:* Slightly prolonged.
- ■ *QT interval:* Slightly shortened. (See *ECG effects of class II antiarrhythmics.*)

Class III antiarrhythmics

Class III drugs prolong the action potential duration, which, in turn, prolongs the effective refractory period. Class III drugs are called potassium channel blockers because they block the movement of potassium during phase 3 of the action potential. Drugs in this class include amiodarone and ibutilide fumarate. All class III drugs have proarrhythmic potential.

ECG effects of class III antiarrhythmics

Class III antiarrhythmics—including amiodarone, sotalol, and ibutilide—affect the cardiac cycle and cause the effects shown here on an electrocardiogram (ECG). Class III antiarrhythmics:
- block potassium movement during phase 3
- increase the duration of the action potential
- prolong the effective refractory period.

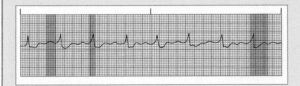

ECG characteristics of class III antiarrhythmics:
- *PR interval:* prolonged (see shaded area above left)
- *QRS complex:* widened (see shaded area above center)
- *QT interval:* prolonged (see shaded area above right)

ECG CHARACTERISTICS

- *PR interval:* Prolonged.
- *QRS complex:* Widened.
- *QT interval:* Prolonged. (See *ECG effects of class III antiarrhythmics*, page 189.)

Class IV antiarrhythmics

Class IV drugs block the movement of calcium during phase 2 of the action potential. Because phase 2 is also called the calcium channel or the slow channel, drugs that affect phase 2 are also known as *calcium channel blockers* or *slow channel blockers*. These drugs slow conduction and increase the refractory period of calcium-dependent tissues, including the AV node. Drugs in this class include verapamil and diltiazem.

ECG effects of class IV antiarrhythmics

Class IV antiarrhythmics—including such calcium channel blockers as verapamil and diltiazem—affect the cardiac cycle in specific ways and may lead to a prolonged PR interval, as shown here. Class IV antiarrhythmics:

- block calcium movement during phase 2
- prolong the conduction time and increase the refractory period in the atrioventricular node
- decrease contractility.

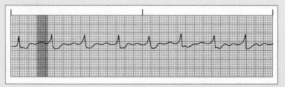

Electrocardiogram (ECG) characteristics of class IV antiarrhythmics:

- PR interval: prolonged (see shaded area)

ECG CHARACTERISTICS
- *Rate:* Atrial and ventricular rates are decreased.
- *PR interval:* Prolonged. (See *ECG effects of class IV antiarrhythmics.*)

Unclassified antiarrhythmics

ADENOSINE
Adenosine is a naturally occurring nucleoside used to slow the heart rate and to restore normal conduction. It depresses the SA node's pacemaker activity, reducing the heart rate and the AV node's ability to conduct impulses from the atria to the ventricles. Adenosine isn't chemically related to any other antiarrhythmic.

Adenosine is most effective in treating reentry tachycardias that involve the AV node. It's also effective with more than 90% of paroxysmal supraventricular tachycardia (PSVT) and is particularly useful in treating arrhythmias related to accessory bypass tracts such as in Wolff-Parkinson-White syndrome.

Adenosine has a very short half-life and must be given by rapid I.V. push, followed by an immediate flush of 20 ml of normal saline. Because of the risk of a heart block, the patient must be monitored while receiving this drug.

ECG characteristics
- *Rate:* Varies—begins tachycardic and becomes normal.
- *PR interval:* Difficult to determine at beginning, then normal or occasionally with a first-degree block.
- *QT interval:* Shortened due to the increased heart rate, then normal when the heart rate slows.
- *Other:* Often causes an asystolic pause, lasting a few seconds, at the time of conversion. (See *ECG effects of adenosine,* page 192.)

ECG effects of adenosine

Adenosine effects the conduction through the atrioventricular node and may lead to the electrocardiogram (ECG) changes shown here.

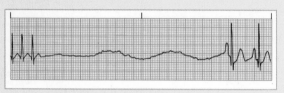

ECG characteristics of adenosine:
- Tachycardia converting to a sinus rhythm
- Short asystolic pause at the time of conversion

ATROPINE

Atropine is an anticholinergic that works by blocking the neurotransmitter acetylcholine. When the cholinergic receptors are stimulated by acetylcholine, vagal stimulation increases, which decreases the heart rate. When atropine is given, it competes with acetylcholine to bind to the cholinergic receptors on the SA and the AV nodes. By blocking acetylcholine from these receptors, atropine increases the heart rate. Atropine is indicated for the treatment of symptomatic bradycardia.

Atropine may need to be given more than once, as the effects wear off. It shouldn't be given for bradycardia in the presence of an acute myocardial infarction. Doing so will cause an increase in the myocardial oxygen consumption and a worsening of the infarction.

ECG characteristics
- *Rate:* Atrial and ventricular rates are increased.
- *PR interval:* Varies depending on underlying rhythm.

- *QT interval:* Decreases as the rate increases.
- *Other:* Causes a gradual increase in the rate.

EPINEPHRINE

Epinephrine is a catecholamine that works on the alpha- and beta-adrenergic receptor sites of the sympathetic nervous system. It increases the force of the contraction of the heart, increasing the heart's workload and oxygen demand. It can also stimulate the pacemaker cells in the SA node to depolarize at a faster rate, producing a positive chronotropic effect. This leads to an increase in the heart rate and also in the blood pressure. Epinephrine is indicated to help restore cardiac rhythm in cardiac arrest and to treat symptomatic bradycardia.

ECG characteristics

- *Rate:* Atrial and ventricular rates are increased.
- *PR interval:* Varies depending on underlying rhythm.
- *QT interval:* Decreases as the rate increases.
- *Other:* Causes a gradual increase in the rate.

DIGOXIN

Digoxin, the most commonly used cardiac glycoside, works by inhibiting the enzyme adenosine triphosphatase. This enzyme is found in the plasma membrane and acts as a pump to exchange sodium ions for potassium ions. Inhibition of sodium-potassium–activated adenosine triphosphatase results in enhanced movement of calcium from the extracellular space to the intracellular space, thereby strengthening myocardial contractions.

The effects of digoxin on the electrical properties of the heart include direct and autonomic effects. Direct effects result in shortening of the action potential, which contributes to the shortening of atrial and ventricular refractoriness. Autonomic effects involve the sympathetic

ECG effects of digoxin

Digoxin affects the cardiac cycle in various ways and may lead to the electrocardiogram (ECG) changes shown here.

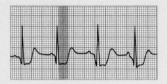

ECG characteristics of digoxin:
- *ST segment:* gradual sloping, causing ST-segment depression in the opposite direction of the QRS deflection (see shaded area)
- *P wave:* may be notched

and parasympathetic systems. Vagal tone is enhanced, and conduction through the SA and AV nodes is slowed. The drug also exerts an antiarrhythmic effect.

Digoxin is used for:
- heart failure
- PSVT
- atrial fibrillation
- atrial flutter.

Digoxin has a very narrow window of therapeutic effectiveness and, at toxic levels, may cause numerous arrhythmias, including paroxysmal atrial tachycardia with block, AV block, atrial and junctional tachyarrhythmias, and ventricular arrhythmias. (See *ECG effects of digoxin*.)

ECG characteristics
- *Rate:* Atrial and ventricular rates are decreased.
- *PR interval:* Shortened.
- *T wave amplitude:* Decreased.

- *ST segment:* Shortened and depressed. Sagging (scooping or sloping) of the segment is characteristic.
- *QT interval:* Shortened due to the shortened ST segment.

Drug distribution and clearance

Many patients receive antiarrhythmics by I.V. bolus or infusion because these drugs are more readily available in that form rather than in an oral form. The cardiovascular system then distributes the drugs throughout the body, specifically to the site of action.

Most drugs are changed, or biotransformed, into active or inactive metabolites in the liver. The kidneys are the primary sites for the excretion of those metabolites. When caring for a patient receiving these drugs, remember that patients with impaired heart, liver, or kidney function may suffer from inadequate drug effect or toxicity. (See *Drug metabolism and elimination across the life span.*)

LIFE STAGES

Drug metabolism and elimination across the life span

Neonates have a reduced ability to metabolize drugs because of the limited activity of hepatic enzymes at the time of birth. As the infant grows, drug metabolism improves. The glomerular filtration rate is also reduced at birth, causing neonates to eliminate drugs more slowly than adults.

In older patients, advancing age usually reduces the blood supply to the liver and certain liver enzymes become less active. Consequently, the liver loses some of its ability to metabolize drugs. With reduced liver function, higher drug levels remain in circulation, causing more intense drug effects and increasing the risk of drug toxicity. Because kidney function also diminishes with age, drug elimination may be impaired, resulting in increased drug levels.

NONPHARMACOLOGIC TREATMENTS

In addition to defibrillation and synchronized cardioversion, which have already been discussed, nonpharmacologic treatments for arrhythmias include:

- single- and dual-chamber pacemakers
- biventricular pacemakers
- implanted cardioverter-defibrillators (ICDs)
- radiofrequency ablation.

These treatments may be used alone or together, depending on which arrhythmia and underlying causes are being corrected.

Pacemakers and ICDs either stimulate or change the electrical impulses of the heart. This action produces distinctive markings on the electrocardiogram (ECG). Radiofrequency ablation is used to destroy a small targeted area of the heart that's causing an arrhythmia. When used alone, ablation normally doesn't have any distinctive effects on the ECG, other than the correction of the arrhythmia.

This chapter addresses why pacemakers, ICDs, and radiofrequency ablation are used and what the distinctive markings on the ECG mean. It also deals with how to recognize and troubleshoot problems.

Remember that the patient's ECG is only part of the picture. Information, such as the patient's medical history, physical examination findings, and additional diagnostic studies, may be needed to confirm an initial diagnosis made based on ECG analysis.

Pacemakers

A pacemaker is an artificial device that electrically stimulates the myocardium to depolarize, initiating mechanical contractions. It works by generating an impulse from a power source and transmitting that impulse to the heart muscle. The impulse flows throughout the heart and causes the heart muscle to depolarize.

A pacemaker may be used when a patient has:

■ an arrhythmia, such as certain bradyarrhythmias and tachyarrhythmias
■ sick sinus syndrome
■ an atrioventricular (AV) block.

The device may be used as a temporary measure or a permanent one, depending on the patient's condition. Pacemakers may be needed following myocardial infarction (MI) or cardiac surgery.

This section examines how pacemakers work, ECG characteristics, types of pacemakers, synchronous and asynchronous pacing, description codes, pacing modes, assessment of pacemaker function, troubleshooting a pacemaker, interventions, and patient teaching.

HOW PACEMAKERS WORK

A typical pacemaker has three main components: a pulse generator, battery, and microchip. The pulse generator contains the pacemaker's power source and circuitry. The lithium batteries in a permanent or implanted pacemaker serve as its power source and last about 10 years. A microchip in the device guides heart pacing.

A temporary pacemaker, which isn't implanted, is about the size of a small radio or telemetry box and is powered by alkaline batteries. These units also contain a microchip and are programmed by a touch pad or dials.

An electrical stimulus from the pulse generator moves through wires, or pacing leads, to the electrode tips. The leads for a pacemaker, designed to stimulate a single heart chamber, are placed in either the atrium or the ventricle. For dual-chamber, or AV pacing, the leads are placed in both chambers, usually on the right side of the heart. (See *Types of pacing leads.*)

The electrodes—one on a unipolar lead or two on a bipolar lead—send information about electrical impulses in the myocardium back to the pulse generator. The pulse generator senses the heart's electrical activity and responds according to how it was programmed.

A unipolar lead system is more sensitive to the heart's intrinsic electrical activity than a bipolar system. A bipolar system isn't as easily affected by electrical activity, such as skeletal muscle contraction or magnetic fields, originating outside the heart and the generator.

ECG CHARACTERISTICS

The most prominent characteristic of a pacemaker on an ECG is the pacemaker spike. (See *Recognizing pacemaker spikes,* page 200.) It occurs when the pacemaker sends an electrical impulse to the heart muscle. The impulse appears as a vertical line, or spike. The collective group of spikes on an ECG is called pacemaker artifact.

Depending on the position of the electrode, the spike appears in different locations on the waveform:

■ When the pacemaker stimulates the atria, the spike is followed by a P wave and the patient's baseline QRS complex and T wave. This series of waveforms represents successful pacing, or capture, of the myocardium.

Types of pacing leads

Pacing leads have either one electrode (unipolar) or two (bipolar). These illustrations show the difference between the two leads.

UNIPOLAR LEAD

In a unipolar system, electrical current moves from the pulse generator through the leadwire to the negative pole. From there, it stimulates the heart and returns to the pulse generator's metal surface (the positive pole) to complete the circuit.

BIPOLAR LEAD

In a bipolar system, current flows from the pulse generator through the leadwire to the negative pole at the tip. At that point, it stimulates the heart and then flows back to the positive pole to complete the circuit.

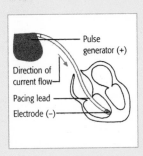

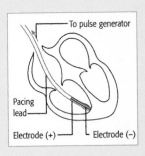

The P wave may appear different from the patient's normal P wave.

- When the ventricles are stimulated by a pacemaker, the spike is followed by a QRS complex and a T wave. The QRS complex appears wider than the patient's own QRS complex because of how the pacemaker depolarizes the ventricles.
- When the pacemaker stimulates the atria and ventricles, the first spike is followed by a P wave, then a sec-

Recognizing pacemaker spikes

Pacemaker impulses—the stimuli that travel from the pacemaker to the heart—are visible on an electrocardiogram tracing as spikes. Large or small, pacemaker spikes appear above or below the isoelectric line. The rhythm strip below shows an atrial and a ventricular pacemaker spike.

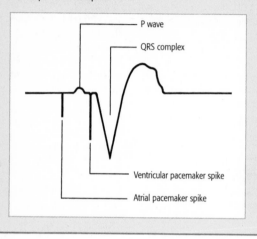

ond spike, and then a QRS complex. Be aware that the type of pacemaker used and the patient's condition may affect whether every beat is paced.

SYNCHRONOUS AND ASYNCHRONOUS PACING

Pacemakers can be classified according to sensitivity. In synchronous, or demand, pacing, the pacemaker initiates electrical impulses only when the heart's intrinsic heart rate falls below the preset rate of the pacemaker. In asynchronous, or fixed, pacing, the pacemaker constantly initiates electrical impulses at a preset rate without regard to the patient's intrinsic electrical activity or heart rate. This type of pacemaker is rarely used.

LIFE STAGES *Older adults with active lifestyles who require a pacemaker may respond best to AV synchronous pacemakers. That's because older adults have a greater reliance on atrial contraction, or atrial kick, to complete ventricular filling.*

PACEMAKER DESCRIPTION CODES

The capabilities of pacemakers are described by a five-letter coding system, though three letters are more commonly used. The first letter of the code identifies the heart chambers being paced. Here are the options and the letters used to signify that option:

- V = Ventricle
- A = Atrium
- D = Dual (ventricle and atrium)
- O = None.

The second letter of the code signifies the heart chamber where the pacemaker senses the intrinsic activity. Here are its options:

- V = Ventricle
- A = Atrium
- D = Dual (ventricle and atrium)
- O = None.

The third letter indicates the pacemaker's mode of response to the intrinsic electrical activity it senses in the atrium or ventricle. Its options include:

- T = Triggered pacing. If atrial activity is sensed, for instance, ventricular pacing may be triggered.
- I = Inhibits pacing. If the pacemaker senses intrinsic activity, it won't fire.
- D = Dual. The pacemaker can be triggered or inhibited depending on the mode and where intrinsic activity occurs.

◾ O = None. The pacemaker doesn't change its mode in response to sensed activity.

The fourth letter of the code describes the pacemaker's programmability. The letter tells whether an external programming device can modify the pacemaker. Here are its options:

◾ P = Basic functions programmable
◾ M = Multiprogrammable parameters
◾ C = Communicating functions such as telemetry
◾ R = Rate responsiveness or rate modulation, which adjusts to fit the patient's metabolic needs and achieve normal hemodynamic status
◾ O = None.

The final letter of the code denotes special tachyarrhythmia functions and identifies how the pacemaker responds to a tachyarrhythmia:

◾ P = Pacing ability. The pacemaker's rapid bursts pace the heart at a rate above its intrinsic rate to override the source of tachycardia. When the stimulation ceases, the tachyarrhythmia breaks. Increased arrhythmia may result.
◾ S = Shock. An ICD identifies ventricular tachycardia and delivers a shock to stop the arrhythmia.
◾ D = Dual ability to shock and pace.
◾ O = None.

PACING MODES

The mode of a pacemaker indicates its functions. Several different modes may be used during pacing, and they may or may not mimic the normal cardiac cycle. A three-letter code, rather than a five-letter code, is typically used to describe pacemaker function. Modes include AAI, VVI, DVI, and DDD. (See *How AAI and VVI pacemakers work*.) Pacemaker rates may vary by age.

How AAI and VVI pacemakers work

Both an AAI and a VVI pacemaker are single-chamber pacemakers. The electrode for an AAI is placed in the atrium. For a VVI pacemaker, the electrode is placed in the ventricle. These rhythm strips show how each pacemaker works.

AAI PACEMAKER

Note how the AAI pacemaker senses and paces the atria only. The QRS complex that follows occurs as a result of the heart's own conduction.

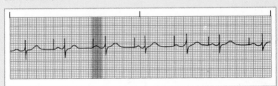

ECG characteristics of AAI pacemakers:
- *P wave:* follows each atrial spike (atrial depolarization) (see shaded area)
- *QRS complex:* results from normal conduction

VVI PACEMAKER

The VVI pacemaker senses and paces the ventricles. When each spike is followed by a depolarization, as shown here, the rhythm is said to reflect 100% capture.

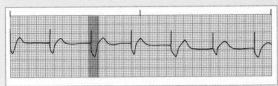

ECG characteristics of VVI pacemakers:
- *QRS complex:* follows each ventricular spike (ventricular depolarization) (see shaded area)

LIFE STAGES In children, the demand rate of programmable pacemakers can be set to a heart rate appropriate for the child's age. As the child grows, the heart rate can be adjusted to a slower rate.

AAI mode

The AAI, or atrial demand, pacemaker is a single-chambered pacemaker that paces and senses the atria. When the pacemaker senses intrinsic atrial activity, it inhibits pacing and resets itself. Only the atria are paced.

Because AAI pacemakers require a functioning AV node and intact conduction system, they aren't used in AV block. An AAI pacemaker may be used in patients with sinus bradycardia, which may occur after cardiac surgery, or with sick sinus syndrome, as long as the AV node and His-Purkinje system aren't diseased.

VVI mode

The VVI, or ventricular demand, pacemaker paces and senses the ventricles. When it senses intrinsic ventricular activity, it inhibits pacing.

This single-chambered pacemaker benefits patients with complete heart block and those needing intermittent pacing. Because it doesn't affect atrial activity, it's used for patients who don't need an atrial kick—the extra 15% to 30% of cardiac output that comes from atrial contraction.

If a patient has spontaneous atrial activity, a VVI pacemaker won't synchronize the ventricular activity with it, so tricuspid and mitral regurgitation may develop. Sedentary patients may use this pacemaker, but it won't adjust its rate for more active patients.

DVI mode

The DVI, or AV sequential, pacemaker paces the atria and ventricles. (See *Effects of a DVI pacemaker.*) This dual-

Effects of a DVI pacemaker

A committed DVI pacemaker paces the atria and ventricles. The pacemaker senses only ventricular activity. The rhythm strip below shows the effects of a committed DVI pacemaker.

In two of the complexes, the pacemaker didn't sense the intrinsic QRS complex because the complex occurred during the AV interval, when the pacemaker was already committed to fire (see shaded areas). With a noncommitted DVI pacemaker, spikes after the QRS complex wouldn't appear because the stimulus to pace the ventricles would be inhibited.

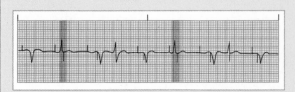

An ECG characteristic of committed DVI pacemakers:
● *Ventricular pacemaker:* fires despite the intrinsic QRS complex

chambered pacemaker senses only the ventricles' intrinsic activity, inhibiting ventricular pacing.

Two types of DVI pacemakers may be used, a committed DVI and a noncommitted DVI pacemaker. The committed DVI pacemaker doesn't sense intrinsic activity during the AV interval—the time between an atrial and ventricular spike. It generates an impulse even with spontaneous ventricular depolarization. The noncommitted DVI pacemaker, on the other hand, is inhibited if a spontaneous depolarization occurs.

The DVI pacemaker helps patients with AV block or sick sinus syndrome who have a diseased His-Purkinje conduction system. It provides the benefits of AV syn-

Effects of a DDD pacemaker

This rhythm strip shows the effects of a DDD pacemaker. Complexes 1, 2, 4, and 7 reveal the atrial-synchronous mode, set at a rate of 70. The patient has an intrinsic P wave, so the pacemaker serves only to ensure that the ventricles respond.

Complexes 3, 5, 8, 10, and 12 are intrinsic ventricular depolarizations. The pacemaker senses these depolarizations and inhibits firing. In complexes 6, 9, and 11, the pacemaker is pacing the atria and ventricles in sequence. In complex 13, only the atria are paced; the ventricles respond on their own.

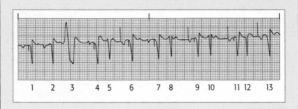

ECG characteristics of DDD pacemakers:
- Complex *1:* pacemaker pacing ventricles only
- Complex *11:* pacemaker pacing atria and ventricles

chrony and atrial kick, thus improving cardiac output. However, it can't vary the atrial rate and isn't helpful in atrial fibrillation because it can't capture the atria. In addition, it may needlessly fire or inhibit its own pacing.

DDD mode

A DDD, or universal pacemaker is used with severe AV block. (See *Effects of a DDD pacemaker.*) However, because the pacemaker possesses so many capabilities, it may be hard to troubleshoot problems.

Advantages of the DDD pacemaker include its:
■ versatility

Evaluating a DDD pacemaker rhythm strip

Look for these potential events when examining a rhythm strip of a patient with a DDD pacemaker.

● Intrinsic rhythm. No pacemaker activity occurs because none is needed.

● Intrinsic P wave followed by a ventricular pacemaker spike. The pacemaker is tracking the atrial rate and assuring a ventricular response.

● Pacemaker spike before a P wave, then an intrinsic ventricular QRS complex. The atrial rate is falling below the lower rate limit, causing the atrial channel to fire. Normal conduction to the ventricles then ensues.

● Pacemaker spike before a P wave and a pacemaker spike before the QRS complex. No intrinsic activity occurs in either the atria or ventricles.

■ programmability
■ ability to change modes automatically
■ ability to mimic the normal physiologic cardiac cycle, maintaining AV synchrony
■ ability to sense and pace the atria and ventricles at the same time according to the intrinsic atrial rate and maximal rate limit.

Unlike other pacemakers, the DDD pacemaker is set with a rate range, rather than a single critical rate. It senses atrial activity and ensures that the ventricles respond to all atrial stimulations, maintaining normal AV synchrony.

The DDD pacemaker fires when the ventricle doesn't respond on its own, and it paces the atria when the atrial rate falls below the lower set rate. (See *Evaluating a DDD pacemaker rhythm strip.*) In a patient with a high atrial rate, a safety mechanism allows the pacemaker to follow the intrinsic atrial rate only to a preset upper limit. That limit is usually set at about 130 beats/minute and helps to prevent the ventricles from responding to atrial tachycardia or atrial flutter.

ASSESSING PACEMAKER FUNCTION

After a pacemaker has been implanted, its function should be assessed. First, determine the pacemaker's mode and settings. If the patient had a permanent pacemaker implanted before admission, ask whether the wallet card from the manufacturer notes the mode and settings.

If the pacemaker was recently implanted, check the patient's medical record for information. Don't check only the ECG tracing—you might misinterpret it if you don't know what kind of pacemaker was used. For example, if the tracing has ventricular spikes but no atrial pacing spikes, you might assume that it's a VVI pacemaker when it's actually a DVI pacemaker that has lost its atrial output.

Select a monitoring lead that clearly shows the pacemaker spikes. Make sure the lead you select doesn't cause the cardiac monitor to misinterpret a spike for a QRS complex and double-count the heart rate. This may cause the alarm to sound, falsely signaling a high heart rate.

When looking at an ECG tracing for a patient with a pacemaker, consider the pacemaker mode, and then interpret the paced rhythm. Does it correlate with what you know about the pacemaker?

Look for information that tells you which chamber is paced. Is there capture? Is there a P wave or QRS complex after each atrial or ventricular spike? Or do the P waves and QRS complexes stem from intrinsic electrical activity?

Look for information about the pacemaker's sensing ability. If intrinsic atrial or ventricular activity is present, what is the pacemaker's response?

Look at the rate. What is the pacing rate per minute? Is it appropriate given the pacemaker settings? Although you can determine the rate quickly by counting the number of complexes in a 6-second ECG strip, a more accurate method is to count the number of small boxes between complexes and divide this into 1,500.

Knowing your patient's medical history and whether a pacemaker has been implanted will also help you to determine whether your patient is experiencing ventricular ectopy or paced activity on the ECG.

TROUBLESHOOTING PACEMAKER PROBLEMS

A malfunctioning pacemaker can lead to arrhythmias, hypotension, syncope, and other signs and symptoms of decreased cardiac output. (See *Recognizing a malfunctioning pacemaker*, pages 210 and 211.) Common problems with pacemakers that can lead to low cardiac output and loss of AV synchrony include:
- failure to capture
- failure to pace
- undersensing
- oversensing.

Failure to capture

Failure to capture appears on an ECG as a pacemaker spike without the appropriate atrial or ventricular response—a spike without a complex. Think of failure to capture as the pacemaker's inability to stimulate the chamber.

Causes of failure to capture include:
- acidosis
- electrolyte imbalances
- fibrosis
- incorrect leadwire position
- a low milliampere or output setting
- depletion of the battery

Recognizing a malfunctioning pacemaker

Occasionally, pacemakers fail to function properly. When that happens, you'll need to take immediate action to correct the problem. The rhythm strips below show examples of problems that can occur with a temporary pacemaker.

FAILURE TO CAPTURE

● If the patient's condition has changed, notify the practitioner and request new settings.
● If the pacemaker settings have been altered by the patient or someone else, notify the RN who will return them to their correct positions. Make sure the face of the pacemaker is cov-

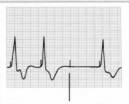

There is a pacemaker spike but no response from the heart.

ered with its plastic shield. Remind the patient not to touch the dials.
● If the heart still doesn't respond, carefully check all connections. The RN may increase the milliampere setting slowly (according to your facility's policy or the practitioner's orders), turn the patient from side to side, change the battery, or reverse the cables in the pulse generator so the positive wire is in the negative terminal and vice versa. Remember that chest X-rays may be needed to determine electrode position.

FAILURE TO PACE

● If the pacing or indicator light flashes, check the connections to the cable.
● If the pulse generator is turned on but the indicators aren't flashing, change the battery. If the battery is functioning properly, the RN or practitioner may need to change the pulse generator.

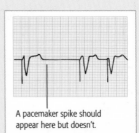

A pacemaker spike should appear here but doesn't.

Recognizing a malfunctioning pacemaker
(*continued*)

FAILURE TO SENSE INTRINSIC BEATS

● If the pacemaker is under-sensing (it fires but at the wrong times or for the wrong reasons), notify the RN who may need to turn the sensitivity control completely to the right. If the pacemaker is oversensing (it incorrectly senses depolarization and refuses to fire when it should), notify the RN who may need to turn the sensitivity control slightly to the left.

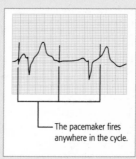

The pacemaker fires anywhere in the cycle.

● Change the battery.
● Remove items in the room that might be causing electromechanical interference. Check that the bed is grounded. Unplug each piece of equipment, and then check to see if the interference stops.

■ a broken or cracked leadwire
■ perforation of the leadwire through the myocardium.

Failure to pace
Failure to pace is indicated by no pacemaker activity on an ECG when pacemaker activity is appropriately expected. This problem may be caused by:
■ battery or circuit failure
■ cracked, broken, or dislodged leads
■ interference between atrial and ventricular sensing in a dual-chambered pacemaker.

Failure to pace can lead to asystole.

Undersensing

Undersensing is indicated by a pacemaker spike when intrinsic cardiac activity is already present. In asynchronous pacemakers that have codes, such as VOO or DOO, undersensing is a programming limitation.

When undersensing occurs in synchronous pacemakers, pacing spikes occur on the ECG where they shouldn't. Although they may appear in any part of the cardiac cycle, the spikes are especially dangerous if they fall on the T wave, where they can cause ventricular tachycardia or ventricular fibrillation.

In synchronous pacemakers, undersensing may be caused by:

■ electrolyte imbalances
■ disconnection or dislodgment of a lead
■ improper lead placement
■ increased sensing threshold from edema or fibrosis at the electrode tip
■ drug interactions
■ depleted or dead pacemaker battery.

Oversensing

If the pacemaker is too sensitive, it can misinterpret muscle movements or other events in the cardiac cycle as intrinsic cardiac electrical activity. Pacing won't occur when it's needed, and the heart rate and AV synchrony won't be maintained.

Interventions

Make sure you're familiar with different types of pacemakers and how they function, so you'll feel more confident in an emergency. When caring for a patient with a pacemaker, follow these guidelines.

■ Assist with pacemaker insertion as appropriate.

- Check the patient's pacemaker settings, connections, and functions regularly.
- Monitor the patient to see how well the pacemaker is tolerated.
- Reposition a patient who has a temporary pacemaker carefully. Turning may dislodge the leadwire.
- Avoid microshocks to the patient by ensuring that the patient's bed and all electrical equipment are grounded properly.
- Remember that pacemaker spikes on the monitor don't necessarily mean your patient is stable. Be sure to check the patient's vital signs and assess for signs and symptoms of decreased cardiac output, such as hypotension, chest pain, dyspnea, and syncope.
- Be alert for signs of infection.
- Watch for subcutaneous emphysema (air in the subcutaneous tissues) around the pacemaker insertion site. Subcutaneous emphysema feels crunchy under your fingers (crepitus) and may indicate pneumothorax.
- Look for pectoral muscle twitching or hiccups that occur in synchrony with the pacemaker. Both are signs of abnormal electrical stimulation and possibly perforation. Notify the physician if you note either of these conditions.
- Watch for signs of a perforated ventricle and the resulting cardiac tamponade. Signs and symptoms include persistent hiccups, tachycardia, distant heart sounds, pulsus paradoxus (a drop in the strength of a pulse during inspiration), hypotension with narrowed pulse pressure, cyanosis, distended neck veins, decreased urine output, restlessness, and complaints of fullness in the chest. Notify the physician immediately if you note any of these signs and symptoms.

PATIENT TEACHING

Following pacemaker insertion, be sure to cover the following points with the patient and his family:

■ Explain why a pacemaker is needed, how it works, and what can be expected from it.

■ Warn the patient with a temporary pacemaker not to get out of bed without assistance.

■ Warn the patient with a transcutaneous pacemaker to expect twitching of the pectoral muscles. Reassure him that analgesics will be given if the discomfort becomes intolerable.

■ Instruct the patient not to manipulate the pacemaker wires or pulse generator.

■ Give the patient with a permanent pacemaker the manufacturer's identification card, and tell him that it should be carried at all times.

■ Teach the patient and his family members how to care for the incision, signs and symptoms of infection, how to take a pulse, and what to do if the pulse drops below the pacemaker rate.

■ Advise the patient to avoid tight clothing or other direct pressure over the pulse generator, to avoid magnetic resonance imaging (MRI) and certain other diagnostic studies, to avoid putting a cell phone close to the pacemaker generator, and to notify the physician if confusion, light-headedness, or shortness of breath occur. The patient should also notify the practitioner if palpitations, prolonged hiccups, or a rapid or an unusually slow heart rate occur.

TYPES OF PACEMAKERS

A pacemaker can be permanent or temporary. Temporary pacemakers may be transvenous, epicardial, transcutaneous, or transthoracic. Certain pacemakers also pace both the left and right ventricles.

Permanent pacemakers

A permanent pacemaker is used to treat chronic heart conditions such as AV block. It's surgically implanted, usually under local anesthesia. The leads are placed transvenously, positioned in the appropriate chambers, and then anchored to the endocardium. (See *Placing a permanent pacemaker,* page 216.)

The generator is then implanted in a pocket made from subcutaneous tissue. The pocket is usually constructed under the clavicle. Most permanent pacemakers are programmed before implantation. The programming sets the conditions under which the pacemaker functions and can be adjusted externally if necessary.

BIVENTRICULAR PACEMAKERS

Biventricular pacemakers provide cardiac resynchronization therapy for patients with moderate and severe heart failure. These patients have intraventricular conduction defects, which result in uncoordinated contraction of the right and left ventricles and a wide QRS complex. Left ventricular dyssynchrony has been associated with worsening heart failure and increased morbidity and mortality. However, not all patients will benefit from a biventricular pacemaker. A patient must have systolic heart failure and ventricular dyssynchrony and these characteristics:

■ Symptomatic heart failure despite maximum medical therapy
■ Moderate to severe heart failure (New York Heart Association class III or IV)
■ A QRS complex longer than 0.13 second
■ Left ventricular ejection fraction of 35% or less.

Placing a permanent pacemaker

A physician who implants an endocardial pacemaker usually selects a transvenous route and begins lead placement by inserting a catheter percutaneously or by venous cutdown. Then, using fluoroscopic guidance, the catheter is threaded through the vein until the tip reaches the endocardium.

ATRIAL LEAD
For lead placement in the atrium, the tip must lodge in the right atrium or coronary sinus, as shown here. For placement in the ventricle, it must lodge within the right ventricular apex in one of the interior muscular ridges, or trabeculae.

IMPLANTING THE GENERATOR
When the lead is in the proper position, the pulse generator is secured in a subcutaneous pocket of tissue just below the clavicle. Changing the generator's battery or microchip circuitry requires only a shallow incision over the site and a quick component exchange.

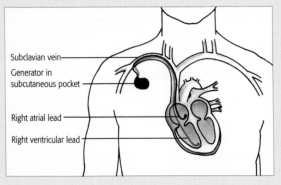

Subclavian vein

Generator in subcutaneous pocket

Right atrial lead

Right ventricular lead

Biventricular pacemakers use three leads—one in the right atrium and one in each ventricle—to coordinate ventricular contractions and improve hemodynamic status. (See *Placing biventricular leads*.)

Placing biventricular leads

Inserting a biventricular pacemaker is similar to inserting a regular pacemaker, except a third lead is placed into the cardiac vein and paces the left ventricle.

A biventricular pacemaker works by sending tiny electrical signals to the left and right ventricles at the same time, ultimately causing the walls of the left ventricle to pump together. The result is more efficient pumping of the heart, improved circulation, and decreased fluid backup in the heart muscle and lungs.

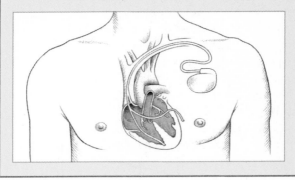

Biventricular pacing has been incorporated into certain automatic implantable cardiac defibrillators and has been used as stand-alone therapy. Much of the care for a patient with a biventricular pacemaker is the same as for a patient with a regular pacemaker. The ECG will show only one ventricular spike.

Temporary pacemakers

A temporary pacemaker is commonly inserted in an emergency. The patient may show signs of decreased cardiac output, such as hypotension or syncope. The temporary pacemaker supports the patient until the condition resolves.

A temporary pacemaker can also serve as a bridge until a permanent pacemaker is inserted. These pacemakers are used for patients with high-grade heart block, bradycardia, or low cardiac output. Several types of temporary pacemakers are available, including:

■ transvenous
■ epicardial
■ transcutaneous
■ transthoracic.

TRANSVENOUS PACEMAKERS

Practitioners usually use the transvenous approach—inserting the pacemaker through a vein, such as the subclavian or internal jugular vein—when inserting a temporary pacemaker. The transvenous pacemaker is probably the most common and reliable type of temporary pacemaker. It's usually inserted at the bedside or in a fluoroscopy suite. The leadwires are advanced through a catheter into the right ventricle or atrium and then connected to the pulse generator.

EPICARDIAL PACEMAKERS

Epicardial pacemakers are commonly used for patients undergoing cardiac surgery. The tips of the leadwires are attached to the surface of the heart and then the wires are brought through the chest wall, below the incision. They're then attached to the pulse generator. The leadwires are usually removed several days after surgery or when the patient no longer requires them.

TRANSCUTANEOUS PACEMAKERS

Use of an external or transcutaneous pacemaker has become commonplace in the past several years. In this noninvasive method, one electrode is placed on the patient's anterior chest wall to the right of the upper sternum below the clavicle and a second electrode is applied to his back (anterior-posterior electrodes). One may also be placed to the left of the left nipple with the center of the electrode in the midaxillary line (also called the anterior-apex position). An external pulse generator then emits pacing impulses that travel through the skin to the heart muscle.

Transcutaneous pacing is a quick, effective method of pacing heart rhythm and is commonly used in emergencies until a transvenous pacemaker can be inserted. However, some patients may not be able to tolerate the irritating sensations produced from prolonged pacing at the levels needed to pace the heart externally. If hemodynamically stable, these patients may require sedation.

TRANSTHORACIC PACEMAKERS

A transthoracic pacemaker is a type of temporary ventricular pacemaker only used during cardiac emergencies as a last resort. Transthoracic pacing requires insertion of a long needle into the right ventricle, using a subxiphoid approach. A pacing wire is then guided directly into the endocardium.

TEMPORARY PACEMAKER SETTINGS

A temporary pacemaker has several types of settings on the pulse generator. The rate control regulates how many impulses are generated in 1 minute and is measured in pulses per minute (ppm). The rate is usually set at 60 to 80 ppm. (See *Setting a temporary pulse generator,* page 220.) The pacemaker fires if the patient's heart rate falls below the preset rate. The rate may be set higher if the patient has a tachyarrhythmia being treated with overdrive pacing.

The energy output of a pacemaker is measured in milliamperes (mA), a measurement that represents the stimu-

Setting a temporary pulse generator

The settings on a temporary pulse generator may be changed in a number of ways to meet the needs of a specific patient. This illustration shows a single-chamber temporary pulse generator and brief descriptions of its various parts.

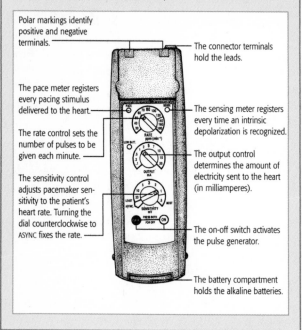

Polar markings identify positive and negative terminals.

The connector terminals hold the leads.

The pace meter registers every pacing stimulus delivered to the heart.

The sensing meter registers every time an intrinsic depolarization is recognized.

The rate control sets the number of pulses to be given each minute.

The output control determines the amount of electricity sent to the heart (in milliamperes).

The sensitivity control adjusts pacemaker sensitivity to the patient's heart rate. Turning the dial counterclockwise to ASYNC fixes the rate.

The on-off switch activates the pulse generator.

The battery compartment holds the alkaline batteries.

lation threshold, or how much energy is required to stimulate the cardiac muscle to depolarize. The stimulation threshold is sometimes referred to as energy required for capture.

You can also program the pacemaker's sensitivity, measured in millivolts (mV). Most pacemakers allow the heart to function naturally and assist only when necessary.

The sensing threshold allows the pacemaker to do this by sensing the heart's normal activity.

Implantable cardioverter-defibrillators

An ICD is an implanted electronic device that continually monitors the heart for:
■ bradycardia
■ ventricular tachycardia
■ ventricular fibrillation (VF).

The device then administers either shocks or paced beats to treat the dangerous arrhythmia. In general, ICDs are indicated for patients in whom drug therapy, surgery, or catheter ablation has failed to prevent an arrhythmia.

The system consists of a programmable pulse generator and one or more leadwires. The pulse generator is a small computer powered by a battery that's responsible for monitoring the heart's electrical activity and delivering electrical therapy when it identifies an abnormal rhythm.

It also stores information on the heart's electrical activity before, during, and after an arrhythmia, along with tracking which treatment was delivered and the outcome of that treatment. Many devices store electrograms (electrical tracings similar to electrocardiogram [ECGs]). With an interrogation device, a cardiologist can retrieve this information, evaluate ICD function and battery status, and adjust ICD system settings when indicated.

The leads are insulated wires that carry cardiac electrical signals to the pulse generator and deliver electrical energy from the pulse generator to the heart.

Today's advanced devices can detect a wide range of arrhythmias and automatically respond with the appropriate therapy, such as bradycardia pacing (both single- and

Types of ICD therapies

Implantable cardioverter-defibrillators (ICDs) can deliver a range of therapies, depending on the arrhythmia detected and how the device is programmed. Therapies include antitachycardia pacing, cardioversion, defibrillation, and bradycardia pacing. Some newer ICDs can also provide biventricular pacing or deliver therapy for atrial fibrillation.

THERAPY	DESCRIPTION
Antitachycardia pacing	A series of small, rapid electrical pacing pulses used to interrupt ventricular tachycardia (VT) and return the heart to its normal rhythm. Antitachycardia pacing isn't appropriate for all patients and is initiated by the cardiologist after appropriate evaluation of electrophysiology studies.
Cardioversion	A low- or high-energy shock (up to 34 joules) timed to the R wave to terminate VT and return the heart to its normal rhythm.
Defibrillation	A high-energy shock (up to 34 joules) to the heart to terminate ventricular fibrillation and return the heart to its normal rhythm.
Bradycardia pacing	Electrical pacing pulses used when the natural electrical signals are too slow. Most ICD systems can pace one chamber (VVI pacing) of the heart at a preset rate. Some systems will sense and pace both chambers (DDD pacing).

dual-chamber), anti-tachycardia pacing, cardioversion, and defibrillation. ICDs that provide therapy for atrial arrhythmias, such as atrial fibrillation, are also available. (See *Types of ICD therapies*.)

PROCEDURE

ICD implantation is commonly performed in the cardiac catheterization laboratory by a specially trained cardiologist. Occasionally, a patient who requires other cardiac

Where an ICD is inserted

To insert an implantable cardioverter-defibrillator (ICD), the cardiologist makes a small incision near the clavicle and gains access to the subclavian vein. The leadwires are inserted through the subclavian vein, threaded into the heart, and placed in contact with the endocardium.

The leads are connected to the pulse generator, which is inserted under the skin in a specially prepared pocket in the right or left upper chest. (Placement is similar to that used for a pacemaker.) The incision is then closed and the device programmed.

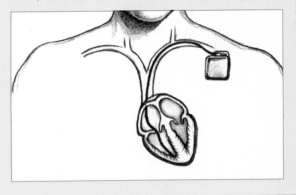

surgery may have the device implanted in the operating room. (See *Where an ICD is inserted*.)

COMPLICATIONS

Complications of ICD implantation include serous or bloody drainage from the insertion site, swelling, ecchymosis, incision pain, and impaired mobility. Other complications include venous thrombosis, embolism, infection, pneumothorax, pectoral or diaphragmatic muscle stimulation from the ICD, arrhythmias, cardiac tamponade, heart failure, and abnormal ICD operation with lead dislodgment. Failure to function is a late complication and may result in untreated VF and cardiac arrest.

NURSING INTERVENTIONS

■ Be aware of how the device is programmed. This information is available through a status report that can be obtained and printed when the cardiologist or trained technician interrogates the device. This involves placing a specialized piece of equipment over the implanted pulse generator to retrieve pacing function. Program information includes:
  – type and model of ICD
  – status of the device (on or off)
  – detection rates
  – therapies that will be delivered, such as pacing, anti-tachycardia pacing, cardioversion, and defibrillation.
  If the patient experiences an arrhythmia or if the device delivers a therapy, this information helps in the evaluation of functioning. (See *Analyzing ICD function.*)
■ If cardiac arrest occurs, initiate cardiopulmonary resuscitation (CPR) and advanced cardiac life support.
■ If the ICD delivers a shock while you're performing chest compressions, you may feel a slight shock. Wearing latex gloves can eliminate this risk.
■ It's safe to externally defibrillate the patient as long as the paddles aren't placed directly over the pulse generator. The anteroposterior paddle position is preferred.
■ Be on guard for signs of a perforated ventricle, with resultant cardiac tamponade. Ominous signs include persistent hiccups, distant heart sounds, pulsus paradoxus, hypotension accompanied by narrow pulse pressure, increased venous pressure, distended neck veins, cyanosis, restlessness, and complaints of fullness in the chest. Report any of these signs immediately and prepare the patient for possible emergency surgery.

Analyzing ICD function

To evaluate the function of an implantable cardioverter-defibrillator (ICD), compare the monitor strips with the device status report. The example shown here demonstrates proper device functioning for ventricular tachycardia (VT) according to the programmed parameters. When VT occurs, the device is programmed to deliver antitachycardia pacing consisting of eight pacing stimuli six separate times. If the arrhythmia doesn't terminate or deteriorates to ventricular fibrillation, the device is programmed to deliver a cardioversion shock. This episode of VT converts to normal sinus rhythm with the first cardioversion.

STATUS REPORT

VT THERAPY	1	2	3	4
Therapy status	On	On	On	On
Therapy type	ATP	CV	CV	CV
Initial # pulses	8			
# Sequences	6			
Energy (joules)		10	34	34
Waveform		Biphasic	Biphasic	Biphasic

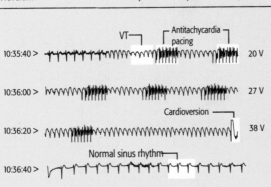

- Monitor the area around the incision for swelling, tenderness, and hematoma, but don't remove the occlusive dressing for the first 24 hours without a physician's order. When you remove the dressing, check the wound for drainage, redness, and unusual warmth or tenderness.
- After the first 24 hours, begin passive range-of-motion exercises if indicated, and progress as tolerated.

PATIENT TEACHING

- Tell the patient to wear medical identification indicating he has an ICD.
- Educate family members in emergency techniques, such as activating the local emergency medical system and performing CPR, in case the device fails.
- Warn the patient to avoid placing excessive pressure over the insertion site or moving or jerking the area until after the postoperative visit.
- Tell the patient to follow normal routines as allowed by the physician and to increase exercise as tolerated.
- Remind the patient to carry information regarding his ICD at all times and to inform the appropriate personnel when traveling or undergoing diagnostic procedures, such as computed tomography scans or MRI.
- Explain that electronic devices such as cell phones may cause disruption of the ICD.
- Stress the importance of follow-up care and physician checkups.

Radiofrequency ablation

Radiofrequency ablation is an invasive procedure for arrhythmias in patients who haven't responded to antiarrhythmics or cardioversion or who can't tolerate antiarrhythmics. A burst of radiofrequency energy is delivered through a catheter to the focus of the arrhythmia or the site causing the blockage of the conduction pathways. Radiofrequency ablation is most commonly used in patients with atrial fibrillation and flutter, ventricular tachycardia, AV nodal reentry tachycardia, and Wolff-Parkinson-White (WPW) syndrome. (See *Destroying the source of ECG abnormality,* pages 228 and 229.)

The patient first undergoes electrophysiology studies to determine and map the specific area of the heart that's causing the arrhythmia. The ablation catheters are inserted into a vein and advanced to the heart where short bursts of radiofrequency waves destroy a small targeted area of heart tissue. Other types of energy may also be used, such as microwave, sonar, or cryo (freezing).

If a rapid arrhythmia that originates above the AV node (such as atrial fibrillation) isn't stopped by targeted ablation, AV nodal ablation may be used to block electrical impulses from being conducted to the ventricles. After ablation of the AV node, the patient may need a pacemaker because impulses can no longer be conducted from the atria to the ventricles.

If the patient has WPW syndrome, electrophysiology studies can locate the accessory pathway, and ablation can destroy it. When reentry is the cause of the arrhythmia, such as AV nodal reentry tachycardia, ablation can destroy the pathway without affecting the AV node.

NURSING INTERVENTIONS
- Provide continuous cardiac monitoring and watch for arrhythmias and ischemic changes.
- Keep the patient on bed rest for at least 8 hours and keep the head of the bed at an angle between 15 and 30 degrees.

Destroying the source of ECG abnormality

In radiofrequency ablation, special catheters are inserted in a vein and advanced to the heart. After the source of the arrhythmia is identified, radiofrequency energy is used to destroy the source of the abnormal electrical impulses or abnormal conduction pathway.

AV NODE ABLATION
If a rapid arrhythmia originates above the atrioventricular (AV) node, the AV node may be destroyed to block impulses from reaching the ventricles.

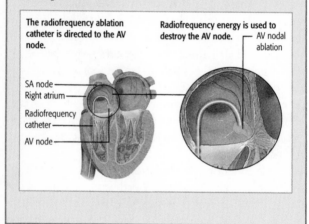

The radiofrequency ablation catheter is directed to the AV node.

Radiofrequency energy is used to destroy the AV node. ⌐ AV nodal ablation

SA node
Right atrium
Radiofrequency catheter
AV node

■ Check the catheter insertion site for bleeding and hematoma formation. Assess peripheral pulses distal to the site, as well as color, sensation, temperature, and capillary refill of the affected extremity.
■ Monitor for complications, such as hemorrhage, stroke, perforation of the heart, arrhythmias, pericarditis, pulmonic vein stenosis or thrombosis, or sudden death.

Destroying the source of ECG abnormality
(*continued*)

PULMONARY VEIN ABLATION
If the pulmonary vein is the source of the arrhythmia, radiofrequency energy is used to destroy the tissue at the base of the pulmonary vein.

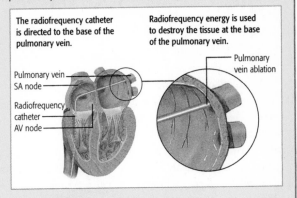

The radiofrequency catheter is directed to the base of the pulmonary vein.

Radiofrequency energy is used to destroy the tissue at the base of the pulmonary vein.

Pulmonary vein ablation

Pulmonary vein
SA node
Radiofrequency catheter
AV node

PATIENT TEACHING
- Discuss why the patient needs the procedure, how it works, and what to expect.
- Inform the patient and his family members that the procedure may take up to 6 hours.
- Provide pacemaker instruction if the patient had a pacemaker placed during the procedure.

10

BASIC 12-LEAD ELECTRO-CARDIOGRAPHY

The 12-lead electrocardiogram (ECG) is a diagnostic test that helps identify pathologic conditions, especially angina and acute myocardial infarction (MI). It provides a more complete view of the heart's electrical activity than a rhythm strip and can be used to assess left ventricular function more effectively. Patients with conditions that affect the heart's electrical system may also benefit from a 12-lead ECG, including those with:

- cardiac arrhythmias
- heart chamber enlargement or hypertrophy
- digoxin or other drug toxicity
- electrolyte imbalances
- pulmonary embolism
- pericarditis
- pacemakers
- hypothermia.

Like other diagnostic tests, a 12-lead ECG must be viewed in conjunction with other data: history, physical assessment findings, results of laboratory and other diagnostic studies, and the drug regimen.

Remember, too, that an ECG can be done in a variety of ways, including over a telephone line. (See *Using transtelephonic cardiac monitoring,* pages 231 and 232.) In

Using transtelephonic cardiac monitoring

Using a special recorder-transmitter, patients at home can transmit electrocardiograms (ECGs) by telephone to a central monitoring center for immediate interpretation. This technique, called *transtelephonic cardiac monitoring* (TTM), reduces health care costs and is commonly used.

Nurses play an important role in TTM. Besides performing extensive patient and family teaching, they may operate the central monitoring center and help interpret ECGs sent by patients.

TTM allows a health care professional to assess transient conditions that cause such symptoms as palpitations, dizziness, syncope, confusion, paroxysmal dyspnea, and chest pain. Such conditions, which aren't commonly apparent while the patient is with a health care professional, can make diagnosis difficult and costly.

With TTM, the patient can transmit an ECG recording from his home when the symptoms appear, avoiding the need to go to the hospital and offering a greater opportunity for early diagnosis. Even if symptoms seldom appear, the patient can keep the equipment for long periods, which further aids in the diagnosis of the patient's condition.

HOME CARE

TTM can also be used by a patient having cardiac rehabilitation at home. He'll be called regularly during this period to assess his progress. Because of this continuous monitoring, TTM can help reduce the anxiety felt by the patient and his family after discharge, especially if the patient suffered a myocardial infarction.

TTM is especially valuable for assessing the effects of drugs and for diagnosing and managing paroxysmal arrhythmias. In both cases, TTM can eliminate the need for admitting the patient for evaluation and a potentially lengthy hospital stay.

UNDERSTANDING TTM EQUIPMENT

TTM requires three main pieces of equipment: an ECG recorder-transmitter, a standard telephone line, and a receiver. The ECG recorder-

(continued)

Using transtelephonic cardiac monitoring
(*continued*)

transmitter converts electrical activity from the patient's heart into acoustic waves. Some models contain built-in memory devices that store recordings of cardiac activity for transmission later.

A standard telephone line is used to transmit information. The receiver converts the acoustic waves transmitted over the telephone line into ECG activity, which is then recorded on ECG paper for interpretation and documentation in the patient's chart. The recorder-transmitter uses two types of electrodes applied to the finger and chest. The electrodes produce ECG tracings similar to those of a standard 12-lead ECG.

---

fact, transtelephonic monitoring has become increasingly important as a tool for assessing patients at home and in other nonclinical settings.

The 12-lead ECG records the heart's electrical activity using a series of electrodes placed on the patient's extremities and chest wall. The 12 leads include three bipolar limb leads (I, II, III), three unipolar augmented limb leads (aV_R, aV_L, and aV_F), and six unipolar precordial, or chest, leads (V_1, V_2, V_3, V_4, V_5, and V_6). These leads provide 12 different views of the heart's electrical activity. (See *Exploring ECG leads.*)

Scanning up, down, and across, each lead transmits information about a different area of the heart. The waveforms obtained from each lead vary depending on the location of the lead in relation to the wave of depolarization passing through the myocardium.

Exploring ECG leads

Each of the leads on a 12-lead electrocardiogram (ECG) views the heart from a different angle. These illustrations show the direction of electrical activity (depolarization) monitored by each lead and the 12 views of the heart.

VIEWS REFLECTED ON A 12-LEAD ECG	LEAD	VIEW OF THE HEART
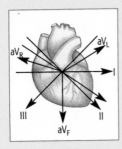	Standard limb leads (bipolar)	
	I	lateral wall
	II	inferior wall
	III	inferior wall
	Augmented limb leads (unipolar	
	aV_R	no specific view
	aV_L	lateral wall
	aV_F	inferior wall
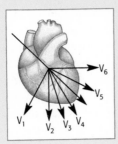	Precordial, or chest, leads (unipolar)	
	V_1	septal wall
	V_2	septal wall
	V_3	anterior wall
	V_4	anterior wall
	V_5	lateral wall
	V_6	lateral wall

Limb leads

The six limb leads record electrical activity in the heart's frontal plane, a view through the middle of the heart from top to bottom. Electrical activity is recorded from the anterior to the posterior axes.

Precordial leads

The six precordial leads provide information on electrical activity in the heart's horizontal plane, a transverse view through the middle of the heart, dividing it into upper and lower portions. Electrical activity is recorded from either a superior or an inferior approach.

Electrical axes

Besides assessing 12 different leads, a 12-lead ECG records the heart's electrical axis. The term *axis* refers to the direction of depolarization as it spreads through the heart. As impulses travel through the heart, they generate small electrical forces called *instantaneous vectors*. The mean of these vectors represents the force and direction of the wave of depolarization through the heart—the electrical axis. The electrical axis is also called the *mean instantaneous vector* and the *mean QRS vector*.

In a healthy heart, impulses originate in the sinoatrial (SA) node, travel through the atria to the atrioventricular (AV) node, and then to the ventricles. Most of the movement of the impulses is downward and to the left, the direction of a normal axis.

In an unhealthy heart, axis direction varies. That's because the direction of electrical activity travels away from areas of damage or necrosis and toward areas of hypertrophy. Knowing the normal deflection of each lead will help you evaluate whether the electrical axis is normal or abnormal.

Obtaining a 12-lead ECG

To perform a 12-lead ECG, you'll need to prepare properly, select the appropriate electrode sites, understand how to perform variations on a standard 12-lead ECG, and make an accurate recording.

PREPARING THE PATIENT

- Gather all necessary supplies, including the 12-lead electrocardiograph machine, recording paper, electrodes, and gauze pads.
- Tell the patient that his practitioner has ordered an ECG, and explain the procedure. Emphasize that the test takes about 10 minutes and that it's a safe and painless way to evaluate the heart's electrical activity. Answer the patient's questions, and offer reassurance. Preparing the patient properly will help alleviate anxiety and promote cooperation.
- Ask the patient to lie in a supine position in the center of the bed with his arms at his sides. If he can't tolerate lying flat, raise the head of the bed to semi-Fowler's position. Ensure privacy, and expose the patient's arms, legs, and chest, draping for comfort.

LIFE STAGES Use patience when obtaining a child's ECG. With the help of parents, if possible, distract the attention of a young child. If artifact from arm and leg movement is a problem, place the electrodes more proximally on his arm or leg.

SELECTING ELECTRODE SITES

- Select the areas where you'll apply the electrodes. Choose areas that are flat and fleshy and not muscular or bony.

- Clip the hair on the area if it's very hairy. Remove excess oil and other substances from the skin to enhance electrode contact. The better the electrode contact, the better the recording.

  The 12-lead ECG provides 12 different views of the heart, just as 12 photographers snapping the same picture would produce 12 different photographs. Taking all of those snapshots requires placing four electrodes on the limbs and six across the front of the chest wall.

- To help ensure an accurate recording, apply the electrodes correctly.

Placing limb leads

Proper lead placement is critical for the accurate recording of cardiac rhythms. The diagrams here show electrode placement for the six limb leads. RA indicates right arm; LA, left arm; RL, right leg; and

LEAD I	**LEAD II**	**LEAD III**
Lead I connects the right arm (negative pole) with the left arm (positive pole).	Lead II connects the right arm (negative pole) with the left leg (positive pole).	Lead III connects the left arm (negative pole) with the left leg (positive pole).

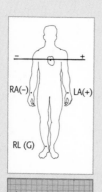 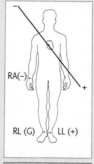 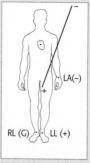

Inaccurate placement of an electrode by greater than ⅗" (1.5 cm) from its standardized position may lead to inaccurate waveforms and an incorrect ECG interpretation.

Limb lead placement

■ To record the bipolar limb leads I, II, and III and the unipolar limb leads aV_R, aV_L, and aV_F, place electrodes on both of the patient's arms and on his left leg. The right leg also receives an electrode, but that electrode acts as a ground and doesn't contribute to the waveform. (See *Placing limb leads*.)

LL, left leg. The plus sign (+) indicates the positive pole, the minus sign (–) indicates the negative pole, and G indicates the ground. Below each diagram is a sample ECG recording for that lead.

LEAD aV_R
Lead aV_R connects the right arm (positive pole) with the heart (negative pole).

LEAD aV_L
Lead aV_L connects the left arm (positive pole) with the heart (negative pole).

LEAD aV_F
Lead aV_F connects the left leg (positive pole) with the heart (negative pole).

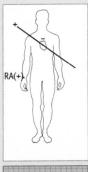

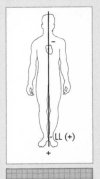

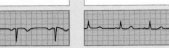

■ Placing the electrodes on the patient is typically easy because each leadwire is labeled or color-coded. For example, a wire (usually white) might be labeled "RA" for right arm. Another (usually red) might be labeled "LL" for left leg.

Precordial lead placement

Precordial leads are also labeled or color-coded according to which wire corresponds to which lead. To record the six precordial leads (V_1 through V_6), position the electrodes on specific areas of the anterior chest wall. (See *Placing precordial leads.*) If they're placed too low or too high, the ECG tracing will be inaccurate.

■ Place lead V_1 over the fourth intercostal space at the right sternal border. To find the space, locate the sternal notch at the second rib and feel your way down the sternal border until you reach the fourth intercostal space.

■ Place lead V_2 just opposite V_1, over the fourth intercostal space at the left sternal border.

■ Place lead V_4 over the fifth intercostal space at the left midclavicular line. Placing lead V_4 before V_3 makes it easier to see where to place lead V_3.

■ Place lead V_3 midway between V_2 and V_4.

■ Place lead V_5 over the fifth intercostal space at the left anterior axillary line.

■ Place lead V_6 over the fifth intercostal space at the left midaxillary line. If you've placed leads V_4 through V_6 correctly, they should line up horizontally.

ADDITIONAL TYPES OF ECGS

In addition to the standard 12-lead ECG, two other types of ECGs may be used for diagnostic purposes: the posterior-lead ECG and the right chest lead ECG.

Placing precordial leads

The precordial leads complement the limb leads to provide a complete view of the heart. To record the precordial leads, place the electrodes as shown.

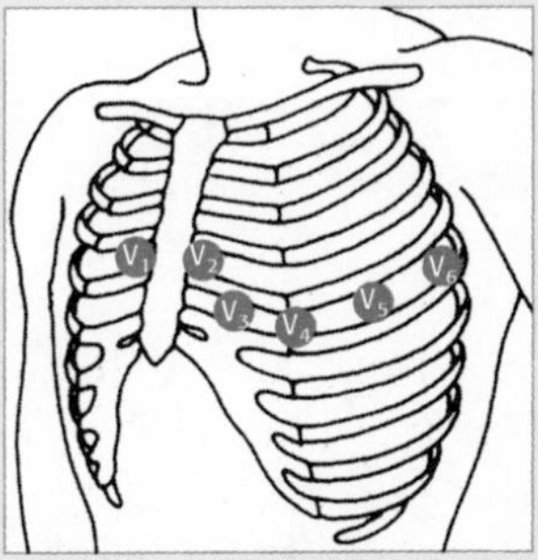

V₁

V₂

V₃

V₄

V₅

V₆

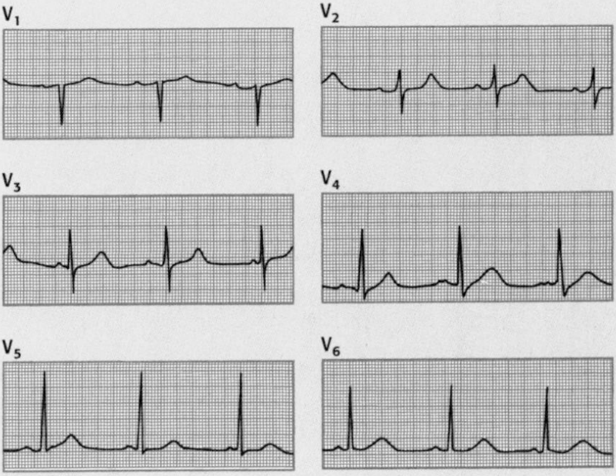

These ECGs use chest leads to assess areas that standard 12-lead ECGs can't.

Posterior-lead ECG

Because of lung and muscle barriers, the usual chest leads can't "see" the heart's posterior surface to record myocardial damage there. So some practitioners add three posterior leads to the 12-lead ECG: leads V_7, V_8, and V_9. These leads are placed at the same level horizontally as the lead V_6 lead at the fifth intercostal space, as shown below.

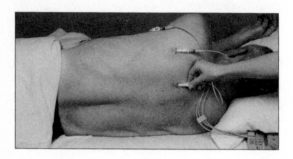

- Place V_7 at the posterior axillary line.
- Place V_9 at the paraspinal line. Placing lead V_9 before V_8 makes it easier to see where to place lead V_8.
- Place V_8 halfway between leads V_7 and V_9.

Occasionally, a practitioner may request right-sided posterior leads. These leads are labeled V_{7R}, V_{8R}, and V_{9R} and are placed on the right side of the patient's back. Their placement is a mirror image of the electrodes on the left side of the back. This type of ECG provides information on the right posterior area of the heart.

Right chest lead ECG

The standard 12-lead ECG evaluates only the left ventricle. If the right ventricle needs to be assessed for damage or dysfunction, the practitoner may order a right chest lead ECG. For example, a patient with an inferior wall MI might have a right chest lead ECG to rule out right ventricular involvement.

With this type of ECG, the six leads are placed on the right side of the chest in a mirror image of the standard precordial lead placement, as shown top of next page

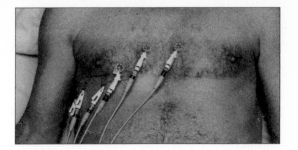

Electrodes start at the left sternal border and swing down under the right breast area.

■ Place lead V_{1R} over the fourth intercostal space at the left sternal border. To find the space, locate the sternal notch at the second rib and feel your way down the sternal border until you reach the fourth intercostal space.

■ Place lead V_{2R} just opposite V_1, over the fourth intercostal space at the right sternal border.

■ Place lead V_{4R} over the fifth intercostal space at the right midclavicular line. Placing lead V_{4R} before V_{3R} makes it easier to see where to place lead V_{3R}.

■ Place lead V_{3R} midway between V_{2R} and V_{4R}.

■ Place lead V_{5R} over the fifth intercostal space at the right anterior axillary line.

■ Place lead V_{6R} over the fifth intercostal space at the right midaxillary line. If you've placed leads V_{4R} through V_{6R} correctly, they should line up horizontally.

RECORDING THE ECG

After properly placing the electrodes, record the ECG. Electrocardiograph machines come in two types: multichannel recorders and single-channel recorders (rarely used). With a multichannel recorder, all electrodes are attached to the patient at once and the machine prints a simultaneous view of all leads. With a single-channel recorder, one lead at a time is recorded in a short strip by attaching and removing electrodes and stopping and starting the tracing each time.

To record a multichannel ECG, follow these steps:

■ Plug the cord of the ECG machine into a grounded outlet and turn it on. If the machine operates on a charged battery, it may not need to be plugged in.

■ Enter the patient information, such as name and identification number, into the machine.

■ Place the electrodes on the patient's limbs and chest.

RED FLAG *Be sure to place the chest electrodes below a woman's breast. In a large-breasted woman, you may need to move her breast to the side.*

■ Make sure all leads are securely attached.

■ Instruct the patient to relax, lie still, and breathe normally. Ask him not to talk during the recording, to prevent distortion of the ECG tracing.

■ Make sure the ECG paper speed selector is set to 25 mm/second and that all 12-lead tracings appear in the view screen.

■ Press the auto button and record the ECG.

■ Observe the quality of the tracing. When the machine finishes the recording, turn it off.

■ Remove the electrodes, and clean the patient's skin.

DOCUMENTING THE ECG TRACING

ECG tracings from a multichannel machine will show the patient's name and room number and, possibly, his medical record number. At the top of the printout, you'll see the patient's heart rate and wave durations, measured in seconds. (See *Interpreting a multichannel ECG tracing.*)

Some machines are capable of recording ST-segment elevation and depression. The name of the lead will appear next to each 6-second strip.

Interpreting a multichannel ECG recording

The top of a 12-lead ECG recording usually shows patient identification information along with an interpretation by the machine. A rhythm strip is commonly included at the bottom of the recording.

STANDARDIZATION
Look for standardization marks on the recording, normally 10 small squares high. If the patient has high voltage complexes, the marks will be half as high. You'll also notice that lead markers separate the lead recordings on the paper and that each lead is labeled.

Familiarize yourself with the order in which the leads are arranged on an ECG tracing. Getting accustomed to the layout of the tracing will help you interpret the ECG more quickly and accurately.

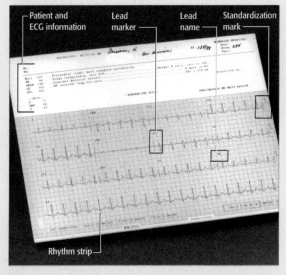

Patient and ECG information — Lead marker — Lead name — Standardization mark

Rhythm strip

Write the following information on the printout: date, time, practitioner's name, and special circumstances. For example, you might record:

- an episode of chest pain
- abnormal electrolyte levels
- related drug treatment
- abnormal placement of the electrodes
- the presence of an artificial pacemaker and whether a magnet was used while the ECG was obtained.

Remember, ECGs are legal documents. They belong in the patient's medical record and must be saved for future reference and comparison with baseline strips.

Ambulatory electrocardiography

Monitoring the electrical activity of the heart while a patient goes about his normal daily routine may provide valuable information to the practitioner. Many arrhythmias only occur during certain activities such as eating, exercise, emotional stress, having a bowel movement, or even sleeping. Because of this, it may be difficult to record an arrhythmia with a standard 12-lead ECG.

In addition to arrhythmia detection, ambulatory electrocardiography (AECG) may be done:

- to evaluate chest pain
- to evaluate cardiac status after an acute MI or after a pacemaker or implantable cardioverter defibrillator implantation
- to evaluate the effectiveness of antiarrhythmic drug therapy
- to assess and correlate dyspnea, central nervous system (CNS) symptoms (such as syncope and light-headedness), and palpitations with actual cardiac events and the patient's activities.

Two types of ambulatory ECG recorders are used, continuous or intermittent. Continuous recorders are typically used for a limited time period, usually 1 to 3 days. Intermittent recorders may be used for weeks or months and are only activated by a patient in response to symptoms.

CONTINUOUS AECG RECORDING

Also called *Holter monitoring,* continuous AECG involves the constant recording of heart activity over a 24-to-72 hour period as the patient follows his normal routine. Some monitors can record heart rhythms up to 7 days.

During the monitoring period, the patient wears a small battery-powered digital recording device that's connected to electrodes placed on his chest. The number of electrodes placed depends on the model that's used. Some monitors require only three electrodes and others require five to seven. The patient must also keep a diary of his activities and associated symptoms. After the recording period, a computer and a cardiologist analyze the information to correlate cardiac irregularities, such as arrhythmias and ST-segment changes, with the activities noted in the patient's diary.

INTERMITTENT AECG RECORDING

Another kind of AECG monitoring is intermittent recording. This type of recording is usually chosen when symptoms or arrhythmias don't occur very often. There are two types of intermittent recorders, loop recorders and event recorders.

Loop recorder

Loop recorders record the ECG in a continuous manner but store only a brief segment of the actual ECG recording in its memory when the patient activates the event marker by pressing a button. Electrodes are attached to the patient's chest as they are in Holter monitoring; however, the patient must start the recorder when he has symptoms. If he loses consciousness, he can start the recorder as soon as he wakes up.

Some loop recorders can be implanted under the skin in the upper chest area for long term recordings. During or immediately after a symptom such as dizziness or fainting, the patient places a pager-sized device over the implanted monitor to capture and save the data.

Event recorder

An event recorder is used only when symptoms occur. One type of recorder requires the patient to wear it on his wrist and press a button when symptoms occur. A second type of device, about the size of a credit card, is carried by the patient in a location where he can reach it quickly. When symptoms occur, he must place the back of the device firmly against his chest and press the start button. The electrodes on the back of the recorder sense the electrical activity and record it. The patient can then transmit the information across phone lines for evaluation.

Signal-averaged ECG

Although a standard 12-lead ECG is obtained on most patients, some may benefit from obtaining a signal-averaged ECG. This simple, noninvasive test helps identify patients at risk for sudden death from sustained ventricular tachycardia.

The test uses a computer to identify late electrical potentials—tiny impulses that follow normal depolarization. A standard 12-lead ECG can't detect late electrical potentials. Patients prone to ventricular tachycardia—those

Placing electrodes for a signal-averaged ECG

Positioning electrodes for a signal-averaged electrocardiogram (ECG) is much different than for a 12-lead ECG. Here's one method:

1. Place the positive X electrode at the left fourth intercostal space, midaxillary line.
2. Place the negative X electrode at the right fourth intercostal space, midaxillary line.
3. Place the positive Y electrode at the left iliac crest.
4. Place the negative Y electrode at the superior aspect of the manubrium of the sternum.
5. Place the positive Z electrode at the fourth intercostal space, left of the sternum.
6. Place the ground (G) on the lower right at the eighth rib.
7. Reposition the patient on his side, or have him sit forward. Then place the negative Z electrode on his back (not shown),

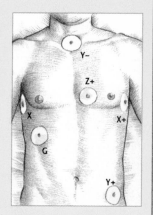

directly posterior to the positive Z electrode.
8. Attach all the leads to the electrodes, being careful not to dislodge the posterior lead. Now, you can obtain the tracing.

who have had a recent MI or unexplained syncope, for example—are good candidates for a signal-averaged ECG. Remember that 12-lead ECGs should be done when the patient is free from arrhythmias.

A signal-averaged ECG is a noise-free, surface ECG recording taken from three specialized leads for several hundred heartbeats. (See *Placing electrodes for a signal-averaged ECG.*) The test takes about 10 minutes. The machine's computer detects late electrical potentials and then enlarges them so they're recognizable. The electrodes for a signal-averaged ECG are labeled X–, X+, Y–, Y+, Z–, Z+, and ground.

The machine averages signals from these leads to produce one representative QRS complex without artifact. The process cancels out noise, electrical impulses that don't occur as a repetitious pattern or with the same consistent timing as the QRS complex. With noise filtered out, late electrical potentials can be detected. Muscle noise can't be filtered, so the patient must lie still for the test.

Practice strips

Use these sample rhythm strips as a practical way to sharpen your ECG interpretation skills. Record the rhythm, rate, and waveform characteristics in the blank spaces provided, and then compare your findings with the answers provided on page 255.

1

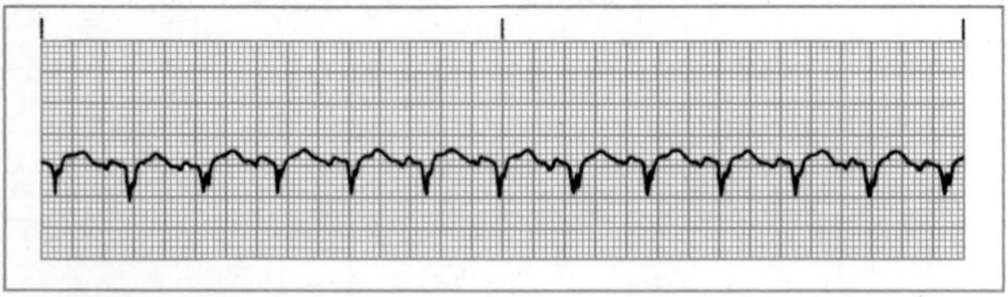

Rhythm: _____

Rate: _____

P wave: _____

PR interval: _____

QRS complex: _____

T wave: _____

QT interval: _____

Other: _____

Interpretation: ___Sinus Tachycardia___

2

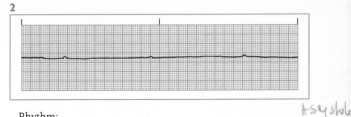

Rhythm: _____ *Asystole*

Rate: _____

P wave: _____

PR interval: _____

QRS complex: _____

T wave: _____

QT interval: _____

Other: _____

Interpretation: _____

3

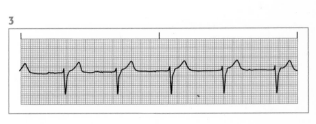

Rhythm: _____

Rate: _____

P wave: _____

PR interval: _____

QRS complex: _____

T wave: _____

QT interval: _____

Other: _____

Interpretation: _____

Accelerated idioventricular rhythm

4

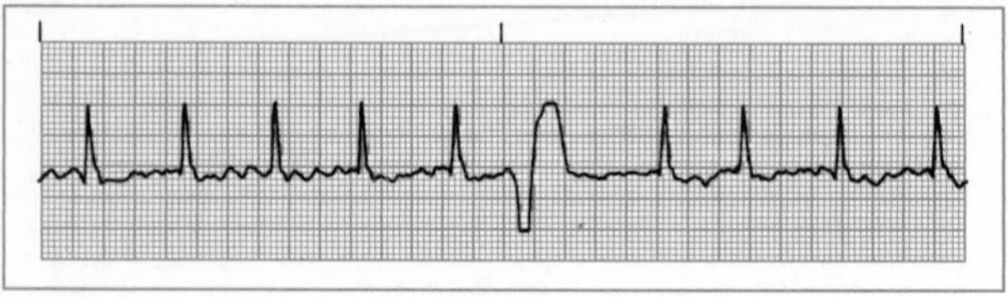

Rhythm: _____

Rate: _____

P wave: _____

PR interval: _____

QRS complex: _____

T wave: _____

QT interval: _____

Other: _____

Interpretation: _____

Atrial flutter w̄ pvc

5

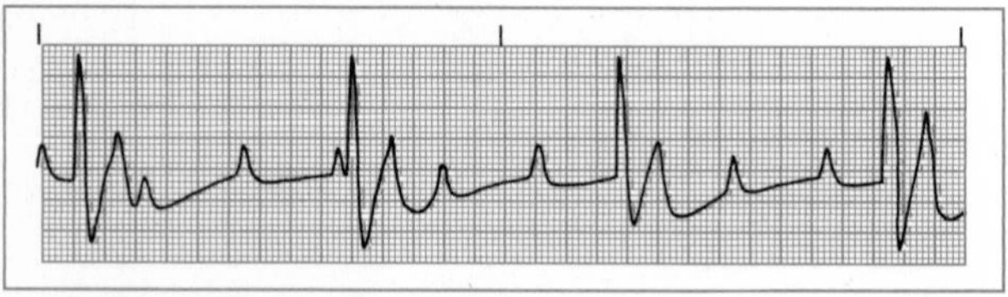

Rhythm: _____

Rate: _____

P wave: _____

PR interval: _____

QRS complex: _____

T wave: _____

QT interval: _____

Other: _____

Interpretation: _____

3° AV

6

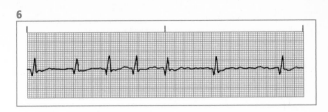

Rhythm: _____

Rate: _____

P wave: _____

PR interval: _____

QRS complex: _____

T wave: _____

QT interval: _____

Other: _____

Interpretation: _____

Atrial Fibrillation

7

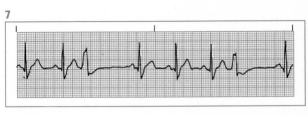

Rhythm: _____

Rate: _____

P wave: _____

PR interval: _____

QRS complex: _____

T wave: _____

QT interval: _____

Other: _____

Interpretation: _____

Sinus rhythm c̄ 2 PVCs

8

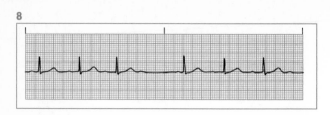

Rhythm: _____

Rate: _____

P wave: _____

PR interval: _____

QRS complex: _____

T wave: _____

QT interval: _____

Other: _____

Interpretation: _____

2° AV type 2 (Mobitz I)

9

Rhythm: _____

Rate: _____

P wave: _____

PR interval: _____

QRS complex: _____

T wave: _____

QT interval: _____

Other: _____

Interpretation: _____

Torsade de pointes

10

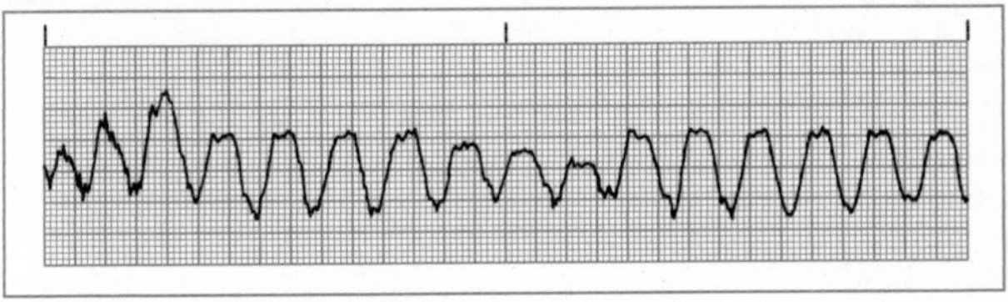

Rhythm: _Irregular_

Rate: _150 BPM_

P wave: _Absent_

PR interval: _Not measurable_

QRS complex: _0.24 sec_

T wave: _Opposite direction to QRS complex_

QT interval: _Not measurable_

Other: _None_

Interpretation: _____
                Ventricular Tachycardia

ANSWERS

1. *Rhythm:* Atrial and ventricular rhythms regular
Rate: Atrial and ventricular rates 125 beats/minute
P wave: Slightly peaked
PR interval: 0.12 second
QRS complex: 0.10 second
T wave: Normal size and configuration
QT interval: 0.28 second; shortened
Other: None
Interpretation: Sinus tachycardia

2. *Rhythm:* Atrial rate irregular; no discernable ventricular activity
Rate: Varies
P wave: Normal size and configuration
PR interval: Not present
QRS complex: Not present
T wave: Not present
QT interval: Not present
Other: None
Interpretation: Atrial activity with ventricular standstill

3. *Rhythm:* Ventricular rhythm regular; P wave not present with each QRS
Rate: Ventricular rate 52 beats/minute; not able to determine atrial rate
P wave: Normal configuration when present
PR interval: 0.32 second
QRS complex: 0.14 second; wide
T wave: Slightly peaked
QT interval: 0.44 seconds
Other: ST elevation present
Interpretation: Accelerated idioventricular rhythm

4. *Rhythm:* Atrial rhythm is regular; ventricular rhythm irregular
Rate: Atrial rate 500 beats/minute; ventricular rate 94 beats/minute
P wave: Sawtooth pattern; flutter waves
PR interval: Not measurable
QRS complex: Normal duration; one aberrant complex with opposite deflection of QRS complex and T wave
T wave: Not identifiable
QT interval: Not measurable
Other: None
Interpretation: Atrial flutter with one premature ventricular contraction (PVC)

5. *Rhythm:* Atrial and ventricular rhythms regular
Rate: Atrial rate 94 beats/minute; ventricular rate 34 beats/minute
P wave: Slightly peaked shape; no constant relationship to the QRS complex
PR interval: Not applicable
QRS complex: 0.20 second; wide and bizarre
T wave: Fourth complex distorted by P wave; other complexes with varied appearance
QT interval: 0.40 second
Other: None
Interpretation: Third-degree heart block (complete heart block)

6. *Rhythm:* Atrial and ventricular rhythms irregular
Rate: Atrial rate can't be determined; ventricular rate varies
P wave: Absent; coarse fibrilliform waves present
PR interval: Indiscernible
QRS complex: 0.12 second; normal configuration
T wave: Indiscernible
QT interval: Not measurable
Other: None
Interpretation: Atrial fibrillation

7. *Rhythm:* Atrial and ventricular rhythms regular; compensatory pause present after wide, bizarre beats
Rate: 75 beats/minute
P wave: Normal size and configuration
PR interval: 0.20 second
QRS complex: 0.14 second, normal size and configuration; third and seventh beat 0.16 second with bizarre, opposite configuration
T wave: Normal configuration
QT interval: 0.40 second
Other: None
Interpretation: Sinus rhythm with two PVCs

8. *Rhythm:* Atrial rate irregular; ventricular rate irregular
Rate: Atrial rate 75 beats/minute; ventricular rate 60 beats/minute
P wave: Normal
PR interval: Progressively prolonged
QRS complex: 0.06 second
T wave: Normal
QT interval: 0.40 second
Other: PR interval gets progressively longer until a QRS complex is dropped
Interpretation: Second-degree heart block Mobitz I (Wenckebach)

9. *Rhythm:* Atrial rhythm can't be distinguished; ventricular rhythm irregular
Rate: Atrial rate can't be determined; ventricular rate varies
P wave: None present
PR interval: Not measurable
QRS complex: Wide, bizarre shape
T wave: Indiscernible
QT interval: Not measurable
Other: QRS complexes spindle-shaped with phasic variation
Interpretation: Torsades de pointes

10. *Rhythm:* Slightly irregular
Rate: 150 beats/minute
P wave: Absent
PR interval: Not measurable
QRS complex: 0.24 second; wide and bizarre
T wave: Opposite direction of QRS complex
QT interval: Not measurable
Other: None
Interpretation: Ventricular tachycardia

ACLS algorithms

BRADYCARDIA

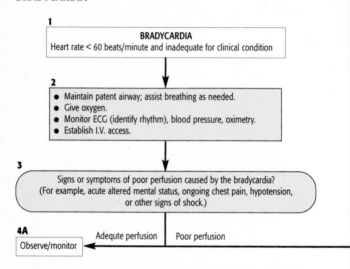

1

BRADYCARDIA
Heart rate < 60 beats/minute and inadequate for clinical condition

2
- Maintain patent airway; assist breathing as needed.
- Give oxygen.
- Monitor ECG (identify rhythm), blood pressure, oximetry.
- Establish I.V. access.

3
Signs or symptoms of poor perfusion caused by the bradycardia?
(For example, acute altered mental status, ongoing chest pain, hypotension, or other signs of shock.)

4A   Adequte perfusion | Poor perfusion
Observe/monitor

REMINDERS
- If pulseless arrest develops, go to Pulseless Arrest Algorithm.

- Search for and treat possible contributing factors, such as:
  - hypovolemia
  - hypoxia
  - hydrogen ion (acidosis)
  - hypokalemia/hyperkalemia
  - hypoglycemia
  - hypothermia
  - toxins
  - tamponade, cardiac
  - tension pneumothorax
  - thrombosis (coronary or pulmonary)
  - trauma (hypovolemia, increased intracranial pressure).

4

- Prepare for transcutaneous pacing; use without delay for high-degree block (type II second-degree block or third-degree atrioventricular block).
- Consider atropine 0.5 mg I.V. while awaiting pacer. May repeat to a total dose of 3 mg. If ineffective, begin pacing.
- Consider epinephrine (2 to 10 mcg/minute) or dopamine (2 to 10 mcg/kg/minute) infusion while awaiting pacer or if pacing ineffective.

5

- Prepare for transvenous pacing.
- Treat contributing causes.
- Consider expert consultation.

PULSELESS ARREST

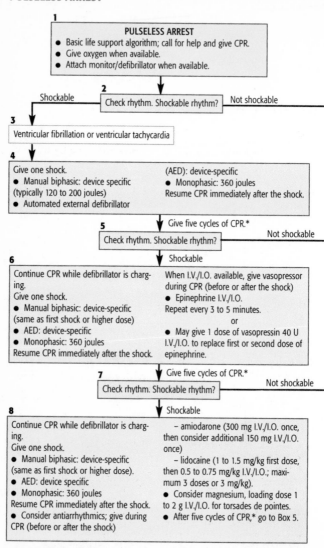

1

PULSELESS ARREST
- Basic life support algorithm; call for help and give CPR.
- Give oxygen when available.
- Attach monitor/defibrillator when available.

2
Shockable   Check rhythm. Shockable rhythm?   Not shockable

3
Ventricular fibrillation or ventricular tachycardia

4
Give one shock.
- Manual biphasic: device specific (typically 120 to 200 joules)
- Automated external defibrillator

(AED): device-specific
- Monophasic: 360 joules

Resume CPR immediately after the shock.

Give five cycles of CPR.*

5
Check rhythm. Shockable rhythm?   Not shockable

6
Continue CPR while defibrillator is charging.
Give one shock.
- Manual biphasic: device-specific (same as first shock or higher dose)
- AED: device-specific
- Monophasic: 360 joules
Resume CPR immediately after the shock.

When I.V./I.O. available, give vasopressor during CPR (before or after the shock)
- Epinephrine I.V./I.O.
Repeat every 3 to 5 minutes.
    or
- May give 1 dose of vasopressin 40 U I.V./I.O. to replace first or second dose of epinephrine.

Give five cycles of CPR.*

7
Check rhythm. Shockable rhythm?   Not shockable

8
Continue CPR while defibrillator is charging.
Give one shock.
- Manual biphasic: device-specific (same as first shock or higher dose).
- AED: device specific
- Monophasic: 360 joules
Resume CPR immediately after the shock.
- Consider antiarrhythmics; give during CPR (before or after the shock)

  – amiodarone (300 mg I.V./I.O. once, then consider additional 150 mg I.V./I.O. once)
  – lidocaine (1 to 1.5 mg/kg first dose, then 0.5 to 0.75 mg/kg I.V./I.O.; maximum 3 doses or 3 mg/kg).
- Consider magnesium, loading dose 1 to 2 g I.V./I.O. for torsades de pointes.
- After five cycles of CPR,* go to Box 5.

* After an advanced airway is placed, rescuers no longer deliver "cycles" of CPR. Give continuous chest compressions without pauses for breaths. Give 8 to 10 breath/minute. Check rhythm every 2 minutes.

Reproduced with permission from *2005 American Heart Association Guidelines for Cardiopulmonary Resuscitation and Emergency Cardiovascular Care.* © 2005 American Heart Association.

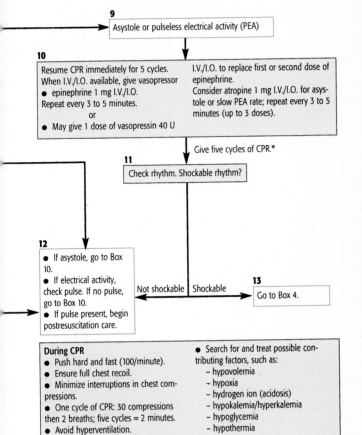

9

Asystole or pulseless electrical activity (PEA)

10

Resume CPR immediately for 5 cycles. When I.V./I.O. available, give vasopressor
● epinephrine 1 mg I.V./I.O. Repeat every 3 to 5 minutes.
                    or
● May give 1 dose of vasopressin 40 U

I.V./I.O. to replace first or second dose of epinephrine.
Consider atropine 1 mg I.V./I.O. for asystole or slow PEA rate; repeat every 3 to 5 minutes (up to 3 doses).

Give five cycles of CPR.*

11

Check rhythm. Shockable rhythm?

12

● If asystole, go to Box 10.
● If electrical activity, check pulse. If no pulse, go to Box 10.
● If pulse present, begin postresuscitation care.

Not shockable ← → Shockable

13

Go to Box 4.

During CPR
● Push hard and fast (100/minute).
● Ensure full chest recoil.
● Minimize interruptions in chest compressions.
● One cycle of CPR: 30 compressions then 2 breaths; five cycles = 2 minutes.
● Avoid hyperventilation.
● Secure airway and confirm placement.
● Rate compressors every two minutes with rhythm checks.

● Search for and treat possible contributing factors, such as:
  – hypovolemia
  – hypoxia
  – hydrogen ion (acidosis)
  – hypokalemia/hyperkalemia
  – hypoglycemia
  – hypothermia
  – toxins
  – tamponade, cardiac
  – tension pneumothorax
  – thrombosis (coronary or pulmonary)
  – trauma.

TACHYCARDIA

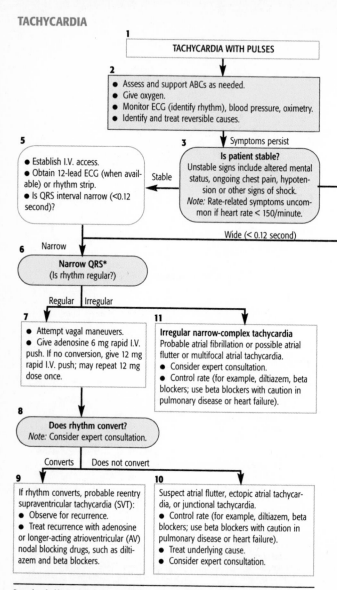

1

TACHYCARDIA WITH PULSES

2

- Assess and support ABCs as needed.
- Give oxygen.
- Monitor ECG (identify rhythm), blood pressure, oximetry.
- Identify and treat reversible causes.

Symptoms persist

3

Is patient stable?
Unstable signs include altered mental status, ongoing chest pain, hypotension or other signs of shock.
Note: Rate-related symptoms uncommon if heart rate < 150/minute.

Stable

Wide (< 0.12 second)

5

- Establish I.V. access.
- Obtain 12-lead ECG (when available) or rhythm strip.
- Is QRS interval narrow (<0.12 second)?

Narrow

6

Narrow QRS*
(Is rhythm regular?)

Regular | Irregular

7

- Attempt vagal maneuvers.
- Give adenosine 6 mg rapid I.V. push. If no conversion, give 12 mg rapid I.V. push; may repeat 12 mg dose once.

11

Irregular narrow-complex tachycardia
Probable atrial fibrillation or possible atrial flutter or multifocal atrial tachycardia.
- Consider expert consultation.
- Control rate (for example, diltiazem, beta blockers; use beta blockers with caution in pulmonary disease or heart failure).

8

Does rhythm convert?
Note: Consider expert consultation.

Converts | Does not convert

9

If rhythm converts, probable reentry supraventricular tachycardia (SVT):
- Observe for recurrence.
- Treat recurrence with adenosine or longer-acting atrioventricular (AV) nodal blocking drugs, such as diltiazem and beta blockers.

10

Suspect atrial flutter, ectopic atrial tachycardia, or junctional tachycardia.
- Control rate (for example, diltiazem, beta blockers; use beta blockers with caution in pulmonary disease or heart failure).
- Treat underlying cause.
- Consider expert consultation.

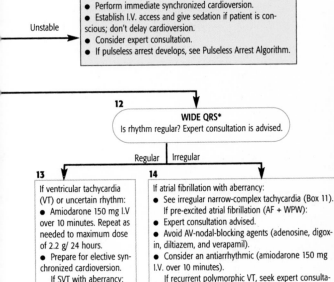

4
- Perform immediate synchronized cardioversion.
- Establish I.V. access and give sedation if patient is conscious; don't delay cardioversion.
- Consider expert consultation.
- If pulseless arrest develops, see Pulseless Arrest Algorithm.

Unstable →

12
WIDE QRS*
Is rhythm regular? Expert consultation is advised.

Regular | Irregular

13
If ventricular tachycardia (VT) or uncertain rhythm:
- Amiodarone 150 mg I.V over 10 minutes. Repeat as needed to maximum dose of 2.2 g/ 24 hours.
- Prepare for elective synchronized cardioversion.
  If SVT with aberrancy:
- Give adenosine.
(Go to Box 7.)

14
If atrial fibrillation with aberrancy:
- See irregular narrow-complex tachycardia (Box 11).
  If pre-excited atrial fibrillation (AF + WPW):
- Expert consultation advised.
- Avoid AV-nodal-blocking agents (adenosine, digoxin, diltiazem, and verapamil).
- Consider an antiarrhythmic (amiodarone 150 mg I.V. over 10 minutes).
  If recurrent polymorphic VT, seek expert consultation.
If torsades de pointes, give magnesium (load with 1 to 2 g over 5 to 60 minutes, then infusion).

During evaluation	**Treat contributing factors, such as:**	
● Secure, verify airway and vascular access when possible.	– hypovolemia	– hypothermia
	– hypoxia	– toxins
● Consider expert consultation.	– hydrogen ion (acidosis)	– tamponade, cardiac
		– tension pneumothorax
● Prepare for cardioversion.	– hypokalemia/ hyperkalemia	– thrombosis (coronary or pulmonary)
	– hypoglycemia	– trauma (hypovolemia).

***Note:** If patient becomes unstable, go to Box 4.

ACUTE CORONARY SYNDROME

1

CHEST DISCOMFORT SUGGESTIVE OF ISCHEMIA

2

EMS assessment and care and hospital preparation
- Monitor, support ABCs. Be prepared to provide CPR and defibrillation.
- Administer oxygen, aspirin, nitroglycerin, and morphine, if needed.
- If available, obtain 12-lead ECG; if ST elevation:
  - Notify receiving hospital with transmission or interpretation.
  - Begin fibrinolytic checklist.
- Hospital should mobilize resources to respond to ST-elevation myocardial infarction (STEMI).

3

Immediate ED assessment (<10 minute)
- Check vital signs; evaluate oxygen saturation.
- Establish I.V. access.
- Obtain/review 12-lead ECG.
- Perform brief, targeted history, physical examination.
- Obtain initial cardiac marker levels, initial electrolyte and coagulation studies.
- Review/complete fibrinolytic checklist; check contraindication.
- Obtain portable chest X-ray (<30 minute).
Immediate ED general treatment
- Start oxygen at 4 L/ minute; maintain O_2 saturation > 90%
- 160 to 325 mg aspirin (if not given by EMS)
- Nitroglycerin sublingual, spray, or I.V.
- Morphine I.V. if pain not relieved by nitroglycerin

4

Review initial 12-lead ECG.

5

ST elevation or new or presumably new left bundle-branch block; strongly suspicious for injury STEMI

6

Start adjunctive treatment as indicated. Don't delay reperfusion.
- Beta blockers
- Clopidogrel
- Heparin (UFH or LMWH)

7

Time from onset of symptoms ≤ 12 hours?

> 12 hours

≤ 12 hours

8

Reperfusion strategy:
Therapy defined by patient and center criteria.
- Be aware of reperfusion goals:
  - door-to-balloon inflation (PCI) goal of 90 minutes
  - door-to-needle (fibrinolysis) goal of 30 minutes
- Continue adjunctive therapies and:
  - angiotensin-converting enzyme (ACE) inhibitors/angiotensin receptor blockers (ARB) within 24 hours symptoms onset
  - HMG CoA reductase inhibitor (statin therapy).

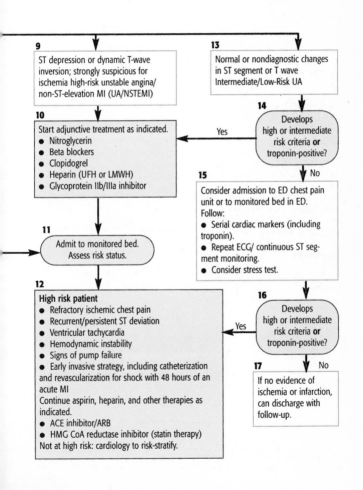

9

ST depression or dynamic T-wave inversion; strongly suspicious for ischemia high-risk unstable angina/non-ST-elevation MI (UA/NSTEMI)

10

Start adjunctive treatment as indicated.
● Nitroglycerin
● Beta blockers
● Clopidogrel
● Heparin (UFH or LMWH)
● Glycoprotein IIb/IIIa inhibitor

11

Admit to monitored bed. Assess risk status.

12

High risk patient
● Refractory ischemic chest pain
● Recurrent/persistent ST deviation
● Ventricular tachycardia
● Hemodynamic instability
● Signs of pump failure
● Early invasive strategy, including catheterization and revascularization for shock with 48 hours of an acute MI
Continue aspirin, heparin, and other therapies as indicated.
● ACE inhibitor/ARB
● HMG CoA reductase inhibitor (statin therapy)
Not at high risk: cardiology to risk-stratify.

13

Normal or nondiagnostic changes in ST segment or T wave Intermediate/Low-Risk UA

14

Develops high or intermediate risk criteria **or** troponin-positive?

Yes → (to 10)

No ↓

15

Consider admission to ED chest pain unit or to monitored bed in ED.
Follow:
● Serial cardiac markers (including troponin).
● Repeat ECG/ continuous ST segment monitoring.
● Consider stress test.

16

Develops high or intermediate risk criteria **or** troponin-positive?

Yes → (to 12)

No ↓

17

If no evidence of ischemia or infarction, can discharge with follow-up.

Quick guide to arrhythmias

Use this guide as a quick reference for identifying characteristics of cardiac arrhythmias. Here are the characteristics of a normal sinus rhythm strip:

- atrial and ventricular rates 60 to 100 beats/minute
- atrial and ventricular rhythms regular
- PR interval of 0.12 to 0.2 second
- QRS duration equal to or less than 0.12 second
- QT interval 0.36 to 0.44 second.

SINUS ARRHYTHMIA

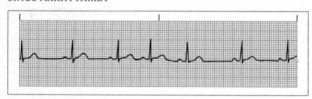

FEATURES

- Irregular atrial and ventricular rhythms; corresponds with respiratory cycle
- Normal P wave preceding each QRS complex

CAUSES

- A normal variation of sinus rhythm in athletes, children, and older adults
- Also seen with digoxin use, morphine use, increased intracranial pressure (ICP), and inferior wall myocardial infarction (MI)

TREATMENT

- Typically no treatment is necessary; may correct underlying cause

SINUS TACHYCARDIA

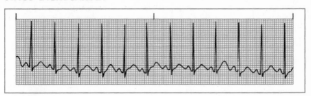

FEATURES
- Atrial and ventricular rhythms regular
- Atrial and ventricular rates are equal; generally 100 to 160 beats/minute
- Normal P wave preceding each QRS complex

CAUSES
- Normal physiologic response to fever, exercise, stress, fear, anxiety, pain, dehydration; may also accompany shock, left-sided heart failure, pericarditis, hyperthyroidism, anemia, pulmonary embolism (PE), or sepsis
- May also occur with atropine, isoproterenol, aminophylline, dopamine, dobutamine, epinephrine, quinidine, caffeine, alcohol, amphetamine, or nicotine use

TREATMENT
- No treatment is necessary if patient is asymptomatic
- Correction of underlying cause

SINUS BRADYCARDIA

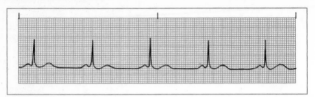

FEATURES
- Regular atrial and ventricular rhythms
- Rate less than 60 beats/ minute
- Normal P wave preceding each QRS complex

CAUSES
- Normal during sleep and in a well-conditioned heart such as in an athlete
- Increased ICP; Valsalva's maneuver, carotid sinus massage, vomiting, hypothyroidism; hyperkalemia, hypothermia, cardiomyopathy, or inferior wall MI
- May also occur with beta blockers, calcium channel blockers, lithium, sotalol, amiodarone, digoxin, or quinidine use

TREATMENT
- No treatment necessary if patient is asymptomatic; if drugs are the cause, may need to discontinue use
- For low cardiac output, dizziness, weakness, altered level of consciousness, or low blood pressure: temporary pacemaker and atropine
- Temporary pacemaker or permanent pacemaker if condition becomes chronic

SINUS ARREST

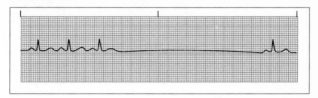

FEATURES
- Atrial and ventricular rhythms normal except for missing complex
- Normal P wave preceding each QRS complex

CAUSES
- Coronary artery disease (CAD), acute myocarditis, or acute inferior wall MI
- Increased vagal tone as occurs with Valsalva's maneuver, carotid sinus massage, or vomiting
- Digoxin, quinidine, procainamide, and salicylates, especially if given at toxic levels
- Excessive doses of beta blockers, such as metoprolol and pro-pranolol
- Sinus node disease

TREATMENT
- No treatment necessary if patient is asymptomatic
- For mild symptoms, may stop medications that contribute to arrhythmia
- If patient is symptomatic, administer atropine
- Temporary or permanent pacemaker for repeated episodes

PREMATURE ATRIAL CONTRACTION (PAC)

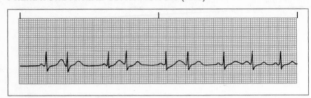

FEATURES
- Premature, abnormal-looking P waves, differing in configuration from normal P waves
- QRS complexes after P waves, except in blocked PACs
- P wave commonly buried in the preceding T wave or identified in the preceding T wave

CAUSES
- In normal heart triggered by alcohol, cigarettes, anxiety, fever, and infectious disease
- Heart failure, coronary or valvular heart disease, acute respiratory failure, chronic obstructive pulmonary disease (COPD), electrolyte imbalance, or hypoxia
- Digoxin toxicity

TREATMENT
- No treatment necessary if patient is asymptomatic
- If frequent, may treat with digoxin, procainamide, or verapamil
- Treatment of underlying cause; patient may need to avoid caffeine or smoking and learn stress reduction measures

ATRIAL TACHYCARDIA

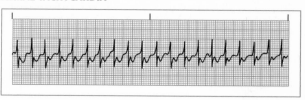

FEATURES

■ Atrial and ventricular rhythms regular when block is constant; irregular when it isn't
■ Heart rate 150 to 250 beats/ minute
■ P waves regular but hidden in preceding T wave; precede QRS complexes
■ Sudden onset and termination of arrhythmia

CAUSES

■ Physical or psychological stress, hypoxia, electrolyte imbalances, cardiomyopathy, congenital anomalies, MI, valvular disease, Wolff-Parkinson-White syndrome, cor pulmonale, hyperthyroidism, or systemic hypertension
■ Digoxin toxicity; caffeine, marijuana, or stimulant use

TREATMENT

■ Vagal stimulation, Valsalva's maneuver, and carotid sinus massage
■ Treatment priority is decreasing the ventricular response by using a calcium channel or beta blocker, digoxin, and cardioversion; then consider procainamide or amiodarone if each preceding treatment is ineffective in rhythm conversion

ATRIAL FLUTTER

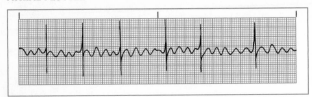

FEATURES
- Atrial rhythm regular; rate is 250 to 400 beats/minute
- Ventricular rhythm variable, depending on degree of atrio-ventricular (AV) block, rate is usually 60 to 100 beats/minute
- Sawtooth P-wave configuration possible (F waves)
- QRS complexes uniform in shape but commonly irregular in rate

CAUSES
- Heart failure, severe mitral valve disease, hyperthyroidism, pericardial disease, COPD, systemic arterial hypoxia, and acute MI

TREATMENT
- Treatment of underlying cause
- Synchronized cardioversion is the treatment of choice
- Drug therapy includes digoxin and calcium channel blockers
- Ibutilide fumarate may be used to convert recent-onset atrial flutter to sinus rhythm

ATRIAL FIBRILLATION

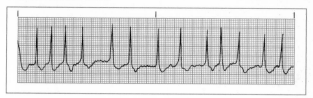

FEATURES

- Atrial rhythm grossly irregular; atrial rate greater than 400 beats/minute
- Ventricular rhythm grossly irregular
- QRS complexes of uniform configuration and duration
- PR interval indiscernible
- No P waves; replaced by fine fibrillation waves (f waves)

CAUSES

- Ischemic heart disease
- Hypertension
- Heart failure
- Valvular heart disease
- Diabetes
- Alcohol abuse
- Thyroid disorders
- Rheumatic heart disease
- Lung and pleural disorders

TREATMENT

- Control ventricular response with such drugs as diltiazem, verapamil, digoxin, and beta blockers
- Ibutilide fumarate may be used to convert new-onset atrial fibrillation to sinus rhythm
- Quinidine and procainamide can also convert atrial fibrillation to normal sinus rhythm, usually after anticoagulation
- Synchronized cardioversion is most successful if used within the first 3 days of treatment

JUNCTIONAL ESCAPE RHYTHM

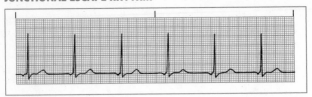

FEATURES

■ Atrial and ventricular rhythms regular
■ Atrial rate 40 to 60 beats/minute
■ Ventricular rate 40 to 60 beats/minute (60 to 100 beats/minute is accelerated junctional rhythm)
■ P waves before, hidden in, or after QRS complex; inverted, if visible
■ PR interval is less than 0.12 second and is measurable only if the P wave comes before the QRS complex
■ QRS complex configuration and duration normal

CAUSES

■ Inferior wall MI, rheumatic heart disease
■ Digoxin toxicity, sick sinus syndrome, vagal stimulation

TREATMENT

■ Atropine for symptom-producing slow rate
■ Pacemaker insertion, if refractory to drugs

PREMATURE JUNCTIONAL CONTRACTIONS

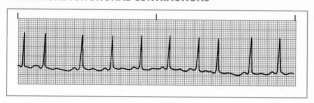

FEATURES

■ Atrial and ventricular rhythms irregular
■ P waves inverted; may proceed, be hidden within, or follow QRS complex
■ PR interval less than 0.12 second, if P wave precedes QRS complex
■ QRS complex configuration and duration normal

CAUSES

■ Inferior wall MI or ischemia, swelling of the AV junction after surgery, rheumatic heart disease, valvular heart disease, excessive caffeine intake
■ Digoxin toxicity (most common)

TREATMENT

■ Discontinuation of digoxin, if appropriate

JUNCTIONAL TACHYCARDIA

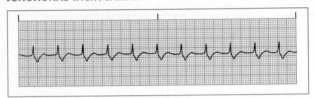

Features

■ Atrial rate is 100 to 200 beats/minute; however, P wave may be absent, be hidden in QRS complex, or precede T wave
■ Ventricular rate is 100 to 200 beats/minute
■ P wave inverted
■ QRS complex configuration and duration normal

Causes

■ Congenital heart disease in children
■ Digoxin toxicity
■ Swelling of the AV junction after heart surgery
■ Inferior or posterior wall MI or ischemia

Treatment

■ Correction of underlying cause
■ Discontinuation of digoxin, if appropriate
■ May require elimination of caffeine intake
■ Correction of underlying cause
■ Discontinuation of digoxin, if appropriate

WANDERING PACEMAKER

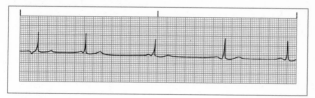

FEATURES

■ Atrial and ventricular rhythms are irregular
■ PR interval varies
■ P waves change in configuration indicating that impulses may originate in the sinoatrial node, atria, or AV junction

CAUSES

■ May be normal in young patients and is common in athletes who have slow heart rates
■ Rheumatic carditis, increased vagal tone
■ Digoxin toxicity

TREATMENT

■ No treatment if patient is asymptomatic
■ Treatment of underlying cause if patient is symptomatic

FIRST-DEGREE AV BLOCK

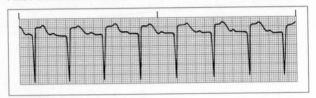

FEATURES
- Atrial and ventricular rhythms regular
- PR interval greater than 0.20 second
- P wave preceding each QRS complex; QRS complex normal

CAUSES
- May be seen in a healthy person
- Myocardial ischemia or infarction, myocarditis, or degenerative heart changes
- Digoxin, calcium channel blocker, and beta blocker use

TREATMENT
- Cautious use of digoxin
- Correction of underlying cause

TYPE I SECOND-DEGREE AV BLOCK
Mobitz I (Wenckebach)

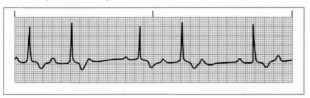

FEATURES
- Atrial rhythm regular
- Ventricular rhythm irregular
- Atrial rate exceeds ventricular rate
- PR interval progressively, but only slightly, longer with each cycle until QRS complex disappears (dropped beat)

CAUSES
- Inferior wall MI, CAD, rheumatic fever, or vagal stimulation
- Digoxin toxicity, beta blockers, calcium channel blockers

TREATMENT
- Treatment of underlying cause
- Atropine or temporary pacemaker for symptom-producing bradycardia
- Discontinuation of digoxin, if appropriate

TYPE II SECOND-DEGREE AV BLOCK
Mobitz II

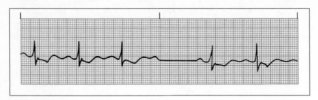

FEATURES
- Atrial rhythm regular
- Ventricular rhythm regular or irregular, with varying degree of block
- QRS complexes periodically absent

CAUSES
- Severe CAD, anterior MI, or degenerative changes in the conduction system
- Digoxin toxicity

TREATMENT
- Atropine for symptom-producing bradycardia
- Temporary pacemaker
- Discontinuation of digoxin, if appropriate

THIRD-DEGREE AV BLOCK
(complete heart block)

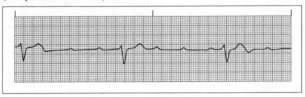

FEATURES
- Atrial rhythm regular
- Ventricular rhythm slow and regular; if escape rhythm originates in the AV node the rate is 40 to 60 beats/minute, if escape rhythm originates in the Purkinje system the rate is less than 40 beats/minute
- No relation between P waves and QRS complexes
- PR interval can't be measured
- QRS interval normal (originates in the AV node) or wide and bizarre (originates in the Purkinje system)

CAUSES
- Inferior or anterior wall MI, CAD, degenerative changes in the heart, congenital abnormality, hypoxia, surgical injury
- Digoxin toxicity and calcium channel and beta blockers

TREATMENT
- Atropine for symptom-producing bradycardia
- Temporary or permanent pacemaker

PREMATURE VENTRICULAR CONTRACTION (PVC)

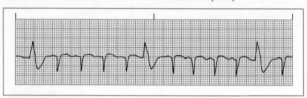

FEATURES

- Atrial rate regular in the underlying rhythm; P wave is absent with the premature beat
- Ventricular rate irregular during PVC; underlying rhythm may be regular
- QRS complex premature, usually followed by a complete compensatory pause
- QRS complex wide and bizarre, usually greater than 0.12 second in the premature beat
- Premature QRS complexes occurring singly, in pairs, or in threes; alternating with normal beats; focus from one or more sites
- Most ominous when clustered, multifocal, with R wave on T pattern

CAUSES

- Heart failure; myocardial ischemia, infarction, or contusion; myocarditis, myocardial irritation by ventricular catheter such as a pacemaker; hypokalemia, metabolic acidosis, or hypocalcemia
- Drug intoxication, particularly with cocaine, tricyclic antidepressants, and amphetamines
- Caffeine, tobacco, or alcohol use
- Psychological stress, anxiety, pain, or exercise

TREATMENT

- If the patient is symptomatic, administer procainamide
- Treatment of underlying cause
- Discontinuation of drug causing toxicity
- Potassium chloride I.V. if induced by hypokalemia

VENTRICULAR TACHYCARDIA

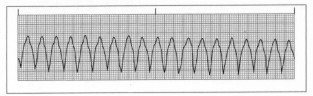

FEATURES

■ Ventricular rate 100 to 200 beats/minute, rhythm is regular or irregular
■ QRS complexes wide, bizarre, and independent of P waves; duration is greater than 0.12 second
■ P waves indiscernible
■ May start and stop suddenly

CAUSES

■ Myocardial ischemia or infarction, CAD, valvular heart disease, heart failure, cardiomyopathy, ventricular catheters, hypokalemia, hypercalcemia, or PE
■ Digoxin, procainamide, quinidine, or cocaine toxicity
■ Anxiety

TREATMENT

■ If patient is pulseless, immediate defibrillation and resuscitation
■ If monomorphic ventricular tachycardia, give amiodarone; if unsuccessful or if the patient is symptomatic, synchronized cardioversion
■ If polymorphic ventricular tachycardia with a long QT interval, stop drugs that may prolong QT interval and treat electrolyte imbalances; if normal QT interval, give amiodarone
■ If episodes of ventricular tachycardia unresponsive to drugs recur, may need a cardioverter-defibrillator

VENTRICULAR FIBRILLATION

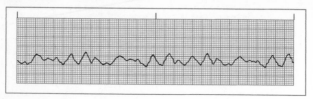

FEATURES

- Ventricular rhythm rapid and chaotic
- QRS complexes wide and irregular; no visible P waves

CAUSES

- Myocardial ischemia or infarction, untreated ventricular tachycardia, hypokalemia, acid-base imbalances, hyperkalemia, hypercalcemia, electric shock, or severe hypothermia
- Digoxin, epinephrine, or quinidine toxicity

TREATMENT

- Rapid resuscitation defibrillation and cardiopulmonary resuscitation (CPR)
- Epinephrine or vasopressin followed by defibrillation and CPR
- Consider antiarrhythmics (amiodarone or lidocaine)
- Treatment of underlying cause

ASYSTOLE

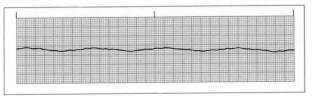

FEATURES
■ No atrial or ventricular rate or rhythm
■ No discernible P waves, QRS complexes, or T waves

CAUSES
■ Myocardial ischemia or infarction, heart failure, prolonged hypoxemia, severe electrolyte disturbances such as hyperkalemia, severe acid-base disturbances, electric shock, ventricular arrhythmias, AV block, PE, or cardiac tamponade
■ Cocaine overdose

TREATMENT
■ CPR, following advanced cardiac life support protocol
■ Transcutaneous pacemaker
■ Treatment of underlying cause
■ Repeated doses of epinephrine, as indicated

ECG effects of electrolyte imbalances

HYPERCALCEMIA

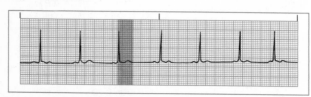

Most of the body's calcium stores are located in bone. The remainder is found in the plasma and other cells. About 50% of plasma calcium is bound to plasma protein, and about 40% is in the ionized or free from. Calcium is important in myocardial contractility, with ionized calcium being more important. Hypercalcemia is generally defined as a calcium level greater than 12 mg/dl.

CAUSES

- Excessive vitamin D intake
- Bone metastasis and calcium re-absorption from breast, prostate, and cervical cancer
- Hyperparathyroidism
- Parathyroid hormone-producing tumors

CLINICAL SIGNIFICANCE

In hypercalcemia, the cell membrane is more refractory to depolarization, which accelerates ventricular depolarization and repolarization. The patient may experience bradyarrhythmias and varying degrees of atrioventricular block.

ECG CHARACTERISTICS

Rhythm: Atrial and ventricular rhythms regular
Rate: Atrial and ventricular rates within normal limits but bradycardia may occur
P wave: Normal size and configuration
PR interval: May be prolonged
QRS complex: Within normal limits but may be prolonged
ST segment: Shortened
T wave: Normal size and configuration but may be depressed
QT interval: Shortened (see shaded area)
Other: None

HYPOCALCEMIA

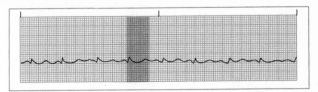

Hypocalcemia occurs when the calcium level is below 8.5 mg/dl and the ionized levels are below 4 mg/dl.

CAUSES

■ Decreases in parathyroid hormone and vitamin D, inadequate intestinal absorption, blood administration, or deposition of ionized calcium into soft tissue or bone
■ Inadequate dietary intake of green, leafy vegetables or dairy products
■ The citrate solution used in storing whole bloods
■ Pancreatitis
■ Neoplastic bone metastasis
■ Decreased intestinal absorption in caused by a vitamin D deficiency from with inadequate intake or insufficient exposure to sunlight
■ Removal of the parathyroid gland, metabolic or respiratory alkalosis, and hypoalbuminemia

CLINICAL SIGNIFICANCE

Hypocalcemia causes an increase in neuromuscular excitability. Characteristic ECG changes are a result of prolonged ventricular depolarization and decreased cardiac contractility.

ECG CHARACTERISTICS

Rhythm: Atrial and ventricular rhythms regular
Rate: Atrial and ventricular rates within normal limits
P wave: Normal size and configuration
PR interval: Within normal limits
QRS complex: Within normal limits
ST segment: Prolonged
T wave: Normal size and configuration but may become flat of inverted
QT interval: Prolonged (see shaded area)
Other: None

HYPERKALEMIA

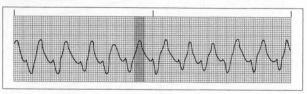

Potassium is the most plentiful intracellular cation and affects many important cellular functions. Most of the body's potassium content is located in the cells. The intracellular fluid (ICF) has a potassium level of 150 to 160 mEq/L, and the extracellular fluid (ECF) has a level of 3.5 to 5 mEq/L. Hyperkalemia is generally defined as a potassium level greater than 5.5 mEq/L.

CAUSES

- Excessive intake of dietary potassium
- I.V. penicillin G, potassium supplements, or banked whole blood
- A shift of potassium from the ICF to the ECF from extensive surgery, burns, massive crush injuries, cell hypoxia, acidosis, and insulin deficiency
- Decreased renal excretion, such as in renal failure
- Decreased production and secretion of aldosterone
- Addison's disease
- Potassium-sparing diuretics

CLINICAL SIGNIFICANCE

Mild elevations in extracellular potassium will result in cells that repolarize faster and are more irri-

table. As the potassium levels continue to rise, the cells lose the ability to repolarize and respond to electrical stimuli. Asystole is the most serious consequence of hyperkalemia.

ECG CHARACTERISTICS

Rhythm: Atrial and ventricular rhythms regular

Rate: Atrial and ventricular rates within normal limits

P wave: In mild hyperkalemia, low amplitude; in moderate hyperkalemia, wide and flattened P waves; in severe hyperkalemia, indiscernible P wave

PR interval: Normal or prolonged, not measurable if the P wave is indiscernible

QRS complex: Widened by longer ventricular depolarization

ST segment: May be elevated in severe hyperkalemia

T wave: Tall, peaked—the classic feature of hyperkalemia (see shaded area)

QT interval: Shortened

Other: Intraventricular conduction disturbances are common

HYPOKALEMIA

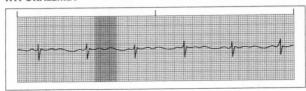

Hypokalemia is generally defined as a potassium level below 3.5 mEq/L. The concentration of ECF potassium is so small that even minor changes in ECF potassium affect the resting membrane potential.

CAUSES

■ Increased loss of body potassium, increased entry into cells, and reduced intake of potassium
■ Respiratory alkalosis
■ Dietary deficiency, most common in the elderly, or in patients with alcoholism or anorexia nervosa
■ Laxative abuse, intestinal fistulae or drainage tubes, diarrhea, vomiting, or continuous nasogastric tubes
■ Diuretics

CLINICAL SIGNIFICANCE

Cardiac effects of hypokalemia are related to the changes in membrane excitability. Ventricular repolarization is delayed because potassium contributes to the repolarization phase of the action potential. Hypokalemia can cause dangerous ventricular arrhythmias and increases the risk of digoxin toxicity.

ECG CHARACTERISTICS

Rhythm: Atrial and ventricular rhythms regular
Rate: Atrial and ventricular rates within normal limits
P wave: Usually normal in size and configuration, but may become peaked in severe hypokalemia
PR interval: May be prolonged
QRS complex: Within normal limits or possibly widened; prolonged in severe hypokalemia
ST segment: Depressed
T wave: Decreased amplitude; T wave flattens as the potassium level drops; in severe hypokalemia, flattens completely, inverts, or may fuse with the increasingly prominent U wave (see shaded area)
QT interval: Becomes indiscernible as the T wave flattens
Other: Increased amplitude of the U wave, becoming more prominent as hypokalemia worsens, and may fuse with the T wave

Best monitoring leads

Most bedside monitoring systems allow for simultaneous monitoring of two leads, such as lead II with V_1 or MCL_1. Lead II or the lead that clearly shows the P waves and QRS complex may be used for sinus node arrhythmias, premature atrial contractions (PACs), and atrioventricular (AV) block. The precordial leads V_1 and V_6 or the bipolar leads MCL_1 and MCL_6 are the best leads for monitoring rhythms with wide QRS complexes and for differentiating ventricular tachycardia (VT) from supraventricular tachycardia with aberrancy.

This table lists the best leads for monitoring challenging cardiac arrhythmias.

ARRHYTHMIA	BEST MONITORING LEADS
PACs	II or lead that shows best P waves
ATRIAL TACHYCARDIA	II, V_1, V_6, MCL_1, MCL_6
PAROXYSMAL ATRIAL TACHYCARDIA	II, V_1, V_6, MCL_1, MCL_6
ATRIAL FLUTTER	II, III
ATRIAL FIBRILLATION	II (or identified in most leads by fibrillatory waves and irregular R-R)
PREMATURE JUNCTIONAL CONTRACTIONS	II
JUNCTIONAL ESCAPE RHYTHM	II
JUNCTIONAL TACHYCARDIA	II, V_1, V_6, MCL_1, MCL_6
PREMATURE VENTRICULAR CONTRACTIONS	V_1, V_6, MCL_1, MCL_6
IDIOVENTRICULAR RHYTHM	V_1, V_6, MCL_1, MCL_6
VT	V_1, V_6, MCL_1, MCL_6
VENTRICULAR FIBRILLATION	Any
TORSADES DE POINTES	Any
THIRD-DEGREE AV BLOCK	II or lead that shows best P waves and QRS complexes

Selected references

"AHA Scientific Statement: Practice Standards for Electrocardiographic Monitoring in Hospital Setting," *Circulation* 110(17): 2721-46, October 2004.

ECG Interpretation Made Incredibly Easy, 3rd ed. Philadelphia: Lippincott Williams & Wilkins, 2005.

Handbook of Emergency Cardiovascular Care for Healthcare Providers. Dallas: American Heart Association, 2006.

Interpreting Difficult ECGs: A Rapid Reference. Philadelphia: Lippincott Williams & Wilkins, 2005.

Jacobson, C.,"ECG Challenges: Tools for Teaching Arrhytmias" *AACN Advanced Critical Care* 17(2):230-232, April/June 2006.

Jones, S., *ECG Notes: Interpretation and Management Guide.* Philadelphia: F.A. Davis Co., 2005.

Index

---

i refers to an illustration; t refers to a table.

---

i refers to an illustration; t refers to a table.

i refers to an illustration; t refers to a table.

i refers to an illustration; t refers to a table.

---

i refers to an illustration; t refers to a table.

i refers to an illustration; t refers to a table.

i refers to an illustration; t refers to a table.

---

i refers to an illustration; t refers to a table.